Healing Without Drugs

A Simple Solution to Your Health Problems

Contains the Essence of Naturopathy,
Water Therapy and Pranic Healing

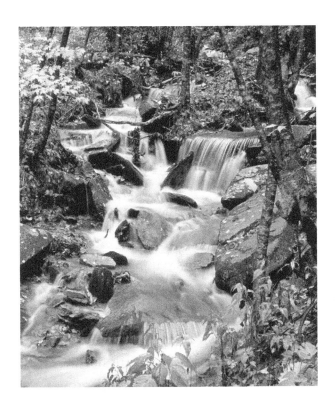

Prashant S Shah

Available from Amazon and Kindle online bookstores

A Disclaimer

The ideas and methods suggested in this book offer you an alternative way of thinking about your health related issues. However, it is up to you make the proper and effective use of them. The author and publisher of this book do not accept any liability arising directly or indirectly from the use of this book.

Contents

A Synopsis **10**

Foreword **11**

By Franklyn D. Sánchez, Ph.D. *11*

By Madanda G. Machayya, Ph.D. *13*

Pre-Publication Reviews *17*

Preface **23**

Introduction 23

How does 'healing' differ from the notion of 'curing'?
.... 26

The basic premise of Holistic Healing 27

A personal note 28

An Overview of the Chapters 30

Acknowledgements... 31

Holistic Healing **32**

1. What are the limitations of allopathic treatment?
.... 32

2. What is so wrong with relieving symptoms? 33

3. What is the difference between a holistic approach
and a specialised approach? 35

4. What is holistic about healing? 37

5. Is there a change in the concept of responsibility?
.... 39

Naturopathy **41**

A. Healing in terms of the vital force 41

    1. What is the cause of disease in the body? 41

    2. What is the vital force and what functions does it perform in our body?..41

    3. What exactly happens when the vital force becomes weak? 43

    4. Why does the vital force become weak? 44

    5. How can we restore the vital force?.....................44

B. Some issues of Natural Healing 45

    1. What is the central idea of natural healing? 45

    2. What happens when we suppress the symptoms with drugs? 46

    3. Aren't germs and bacteria the causes of disease? 48

    4. What is the natural self-healing principle?............49

    5. Which organs of the body perform the elimination function?..51

    6. Do laxatives reduce Toxaemia? 51

    7. Why is the direction of natural healing said to be *'inside out'*?...52

    8. Do medicines cure the disease? 53

    9. What is the effect of drugs on the body? 55

    10. Are there dangers in using drug therapy? 56

    11. When should we take treatment with drugs?.....58

    12. What is the difference between an acute disease and an elimination crisis? 58

    13. Are there other food items that are as harmful as drugs? 59

14. An Overview 60

C. An Estimate 61

1. What is the message of natural healing? 61

2. If natural healing is so simple, why is it not popular? 62

3. What kind of illnesses does natural healing cure? 63

4. Why does modern medical science search only for external cures? 64

The Prescriptions R_x **66**

A. Diet and Eating Habits 66

1. What is the natural health prescription? 66

2. What are good eating habits? 68

3. What is the correct way of eating fruits? 69

4. What is a natural health diet? 70

5. How to adjust your diet to your health condition 70

B. Nutrition 71

1. What is a balanced diet? 71

2. Carbohydrates 73

3. Fibre 73

4. Fats 74

5. Protein 76

6. Sugar 77

7. Dairy Milk 77

8. Acid Food 78

C. Water Therapy 80

1. What is the general idea behind water therapy? . 81

2. What is the nature of the water content of your body? 82

3. What is Osmosis? 83

4. How does the water and nutrients pass through the body? 84

5. What harm is caused by dehydration? 85

6. What happens when the body fluids become thicker? 86

7. What is the difference between acute and chronic dehydration? 86

8. What are some of the usual disorders associated with dehydration? 87

9. Is the need for water in the body regulated by the sensation of thirst? 89

10. How much water do we need to consume every day for rehydration? 91

11. What is provocative detoxification? 93

12. What is 'living water' and 'dead water'? 93

13. How to recognise 'living water'? 94

14. Are there any other properties of 'live water'? ...95

B. Baths & Packs 96

1. Cleansing baths 96

2. Hasty hand baths 97

3. Floating organ bath 98

4. Foot bath 98

5. Wet pack 99

6. Half pack 99

E. The Cleansing Diet 100

F. The Therapeutic Fast *101*
Some additional considerations:........................... 102

G. 'Mono Fruit Diets' and 'Raw Vegetable Juice Diets'103
Mono Fruit Diet.. 103
Raw Vegetable Juice Diet 104

H. The No-Breakfast Plans... *104*

I. Schedule for Implementation *106*

The Hidden Causes of Disease **107**

A. The Stress Factor.. *108*
1. What happens to the body under stress?........... 108
2. What are the physical signs of tension? 110
3. What are the emotional signs of tension?.......... 111
4. What are the typical symptoms of stress?.......... 112
5. How can you overcome stress in daily life? 113
6. Some strategies to reduce physical stress 113
7. How to handle emotional stress? 114
8. Some common lifestyle habits that reduce stress
.... 115

B. The Psychosomatic Causes...................................... *117*
1. Aren't psychosomatic disorders treated by drugs?
.... 117
2. What is the role of trauma in such diseases? 118
3. The psychosomatic causes of certain disorders . 119
4. How psychosomatic disorders are regarded 124
5. Do you have to make some inner changes to
overcome your psychosomatic ailment? 124

6. Can the mind-body relationship be used for self-healing?... 125

C. On handling emotions................................. 125

1. The nature of emotions 125

2. Your interpretations make you emotional 126

3. How to avoid generating personal reactions?.... 127

D. Healing by Changing your Consciousness 127

1. How we become susceptible to disease............ 127

2. The way.. 128

3. Live the truth of health 129

4. A Practice: Choose what you think.................... 130

5. Affirmations for good health 130

6. Some necessary points of view.................... 131

6. Changing the consciousness in organs 132

E. The Karmic Causes 133

1. What is the consequence of a conflict against our conscience?... 134

2. What is the consequence of conflicting with others? 134

3. What is the difference between soul pain and ego pain? 135

4. How can we build our immunity to disease? 136

5. How can we avoid the spread or increase of disease? 136

Pranic Healing... **138**

What Pranic Healing can do for you *139*

1. What is pranic healing? 139

2. The nature of pranic energy.............. 140

3. How pranic energy functions in the body 141

4. What the healer does......................... 142

5. Treating psychosomatic illnesses with pranic healing.. 142

6. The Chakras in Pranic Healing 144

7. The treatment 149

8. Self-Healing using prana.................... 150

Learning to do pranic healing 151

1. Sensitizing the hands......................... 151

2. Sensing the patient's energy field..................... 154

3. Giving the treatment.......................... 155

4. What to expect after the treatment 157

5. How to end the healing session 158

6. Care in discharging the negative prana............. 159

7. Distance healing 160

Appendix **162**

About the Author.. *162*

Other books by the Author........................... **164**

1. The Biochemic Prescriber *164*

2. The Art of Awakening the Soul................... *169*

3. Solving the Problems of Life *171*

4. How to Restore your Health Naturally *175*

A Synopsis

Your health is always your concern and not your doctor's concern. However, today people are made to believe that their health depends on doctors and the healthcare system! It has made the people excessively dependent on the medical profession. And in return the healthcare system has become extremely expensive, and the issues of health have become too technical and complicated for the common man to comprehend.

However, there are alternatives; they always existed! The medical business depends on the progress of modern sciences, but your health does not. You can learn to maintain your health WITHOUT depending on doctors, medicines or hospitals. You do it by simply learning to think holistically and taking the simple self-help measures that can restore your health and keep you healthy. The know-how on how you can do it is adequately provided in this book.

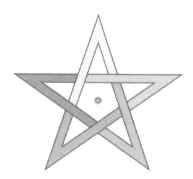

Foreword

By Franklyn D. Sánchez, Ph.D.

Professor Emeritus, Yonkers, NY, USA

This book introduces a very revolutionary concept in health, that by your own efforts you can establish and maintain your health, and that you don't need to refer to doctors, except in extreme cases.

I first met the author in New York in 1994, and I participated in various workshops conducted by him in USA between 1999 and 2013. The general focus of the workshops was on spiritual development. I found him to be affable, soft spoken and endowed with a penchant for humour, usually at his own expense.

During some workshops he commented that illness is really caused by imbalances in the mind and body, and that if we provide the right conditions, he assured us, the body is capable of healing itself.

What are these conditions? Many of us asked such questions. He spoke briefly on the subject, but instead of satisfying us, his refreshingly different view on health and healing generated so much interest that the class pressed him to conduct a full workshop on the subject.

At first he conducted a half-day workshop, then a one-day workshop and then a two-day workshop. Although the workshops were very satisfying, we were always left with wanting much more. We wanted a comprehensive book that we could refer to and recommend to our friends. The present volume has grown out of the exchanges between Dr. Shah and his students. He lays out, in very clear language and in a concise manner, the series of activities that lead to mental peace and renewed vigour. It is an invitation to take charge of your body and cultivate a healthy lifestyle.

Although the language is clear and the procedures are explained in sufficient detail, the major difficulty in applying these principles is the attitude we bring to it. When we get sick, we take out our insurance card and run to the doctor. The doctor gives us some pills, which in most cases relieves some of our troublesome symptoms. There may be side effects, recurrent ailments and even the creation of newer ailments. *But who thinks that deeply?* We as patients do not feel responsible for the ailment in any way. The ailment just happens to us and it is the doctor's job to cure us. However, when things hopelessly don't work out we begin to look for alternative modes of thinking.

This is where this book comes in. It does not talk of curing you. Instead, it tells you how you can remove the cause of the illness in your body and assist the natural intelligence of the body to do the healing. *Why is everyone not doing this?* There is a catch. It requires us to change some of our typical habits, and many of us won't have anything to do with that. However, when we do consent to the change, the results are usually remarkable.

There is much more to this book than I've described. The chapters on psychosomatic illnesses and pranic healing are very unusual and truly amazing. I hope my experience will encourage you to explore this wonderful book.

By Madanda G. Machayya, Ph.D.

Managing Director and Chief Risk Officer, Zurich Alternative Asset Management LLC, New York.

My long association with the author goes back to the 1970's when I participated in his course on 'Man and the Cosmos'. Then he conducted the course through the Indo-American Society at Bombay. Subsequently, in 1980's I moved to USA. Over the years I developed many friends with philosophical interests, and so in 1999 I was able to organise some spiritual awareness workshops in New York conducted by the author. These workshops have continued and are now a regular feature in New York.

In the workshops the author often talked about the 'occult causes' of diseases and the 'law of correspondence' in the cosmos. What I found most interesting was the idea that our ailments originate as a disturbance in the mind. Hence, they can be healed by correcting the thinking, the emotions and the lifestyle, and in most chronic cases medication is not required. We discussed these concepts from time to time and in 2006 the author produced a small booklet on 'Health and Healing'. It aroused so much interest that the author organised workshops on self-healing. The present book is a wonderful write up of the discussions in the workshops and the author has given them an excellent finish.

Another striking feature of the book is 'Pranic Healing', of which the author is a skilled practitioner. I remember an occasion about ten years ago when we were walking back to the subway after a heavy meal, and I was suddenly stuck with a very severe bout of migraine. He asked me to kneel down, and then he passed his right hand slowly over my forehead a few times. We continued with our journey and by the time we reached home about twenty minutes later, the migraine had completely disappeared!

What is really interesting to know is that the pranic healers do not need to know the intricate nature of a disease in detail. They only need to sense the flow of the pranic energy in the body and find out where it is either congested or depleted. The actual process of healing is done by working on the 'pranic double-body'! The author explains this clearly and he also shows how we can develop the necessary sensitivity in our hands to do pranic healing. The amazing thing about pranic healing is that it is simple and psychosomatic ailments, backaches and organ troubles can also be treated in this way.

I've known the author to be constitutionally delicate. He has suffered many repeated bouts of ill health and has also been hospitalised. It was during such times when he was treated and cured, and had to be cured over and over again that he found some basic flaws in orthodox medical thinking and drug therapy. He has explained all this very clearly in this book. However, his aim was not to expose the mistakes, but to find genuine alternatives. And in this effort he went to naturopathic centres, healers and tried out many holistic therapies. He also read extensively on the alternative therapies. He has distilled out the essence and made a fresh, clear and complete presentation of their message.

Many books on naturopathy, water cure and pranic healing are around. However, my impression is that most of them focus narrowly on the methods used without making an adequate presentation of the underlying philosophy and principles that make them really useful. This book has maintained a balance between concepts and methods. It is very well written – the arguments are sharp, precise and striking, and the methods are explained clearly so that they become easy to use. Further, the author has tested the recommendations on himself and others before vouching for their efficacy.

This book is very timely because the world continues to be increasingly dependent on ever evolving generations of drugs. Whereas in earlier times drugs were used only in very severe and acute cases, now they are used to treat every discomfort. The increasingly more hectic and time-constrained lifestyle lived in modern times has created more and more ailments. And these ailments are then treated by more drugs. This has created a vicious circle. Now even minor ailments that can easily be healed by natural methods are treated with pills. However, this overuse of drugs only weakens the patient by increasing the toxin accumulation in the body. Hence, it is very heartening to have at our disposal a very practical set of natural methods that address the root cause of our ailments without creating any side-effects and dependencies. From this perspective, the author has provided an enormous service to humanity and in particular to people who are seeking alternatives to the drug therapy.

Pre-Publication Reviews

By Swati, a Teacher

The most striking point of this book is that the role of the patient in holistic healing is not that of a passive recipient of the treatment, but of a 'participator' in the healing process. The author explains that germs are always present in the atmosphere; however our body becomes prone to disease only when the toxins have accumulated in the cells, which makes them 'ailment prone'. The remedy therefore is not to suppress the symptoms with drugs, but to remove the toxins or the condition of toxaemia in the body.

The relation between emotional disorders and our diseased condition is very well elaborated. I've read such a clear description for the first time in a book. The book is easy to read and there is so much in it that I strongly recommend that you should purchase it. I assure you that you will not regret this decision and that this book will serve you on many occasions, and for a lifetime.

By Sanjeev, a Principal of ITI College

The very first sentence *"Your health is primarily your concern, and not the physician's concern"* conveys the message of book. The modern mindset and lifestyle are such that we do not have the time to take care for our health. Hence, we seek external cures and ignore the inner causes that are responsible for generating the ailments in our body. We like to believe that external factors alone are responsible for our ailment since this absolves us from our personal responsibility. This mistake and the misconceptions that arise from it are wonderfully addressed in this book.

The limitations of modern medicine, the allopathic treatment, are well explained, but the author does acknowledge the usefulness of the allopathic treatment under certain conditions. On the other hand, the author explains the concept of health, the nature of the vital force, and the effect of imbalance in the body very clearly. Further, he shows simple ways in which we can restore the loss of balance in our body and overcome the cause of our ailments. The chapters on water therapy and pranic healing are superb. The information on diet and eating habits is very revealing. I must admit that I've learnt so many things just by reading this book.

The book is not a collection of facts, but it is a brilliant articulation of the experience of the author. And he has written it in very simple language which can be understood even by a layman. The writing is precise and to the point. There is a genuine need for such a book in our society today and I sincerely hope the book will reach the people who really need it.

By Saket, Manager of a software company

Your previous booklet on *Health & Healing without Drugs,* 2006 edition, gave me the message that I have to be more self-reliant in health matters and that medicines are not going to eradicate the root cause of my ailments. By adopting the ideas and methods suggested in that book I've not only reduced my dependence on medicines, but my overall health has markedly improved. And now the present book, *"Healing without Drugs"*, 2014 edition, is two notches up – the usefulness of this book far exceeds my expectations. It builds upon the principles of the earlier booklet, but the descriptions are more detailed and striking, and there are more remedies and many of them are easy to implement. Further, the discussion of emotional and lifestyle causes is very revealing.

In the past I always associated some fear and anxiety with diseases and ailments. My mindset was ingrained with the idea that if medicines are not taken the disease and discomfort would only increase. However, experience has told me that more often taking pills for ailments only complicates matters: It suppresses the symptoms of the ailment giving an illusion of cure; then, there are the side-effects of the drugs, some new chronic symptoms arise, and we get repeated bouts of the same ailment.

Here is a book that will empower you to take control over your health and maintain it for a lifetime, perhaps even without depending upon the medical profession. I plan to gift this book to all my friends and family members.

By Carmen, a retired Government Executive

I have been part of the New York based group that has been participating in the spiritual awareness workshops that were conducted by Prashant over the past ten years. One subject that attracted my interest the most was *'Pranic Healing'*. As a child in Puerto Rico I had seen my mother heal many adults and children just by laying her hands over them. She was a well known healer. However, I didn't know how it worked until I saw Prashant do it and explain it in very simple words. I've seen him scan the body with his hands to diagnose the ailment, pull out the disturbed energy from certain locations, and then gently charge up the person.

I'd like to narrate one incident. My friend has been suffering from urological cancer for over 13 years. During this period he has had several surgeries and has been treated with radiation. In addition, he has to undertake various tests, specifically a body PET scan every three or six months. On October 8th 2013, his doctor told him that his PET scan revealed a cancerous nodule in his groin area. He was told that he had to either be treated with radiation/chemotherapy or have surgery of the affected part. Another test had been scheduled a week later to look at the nodule in a more detailed manner before the treatment. During that time I took my friend to Prashant a few times for pranic healing. My friend was also suffering from '*Peripheral Cardiovascular Disease*' and he was in constant pain and unable to walk more than 50 feet at a time. Prashant cleared his energy blockages and charged him up, and that made him feel really good. However, Prashant remarked that big troubles don't just go away.

The following week, my friend went to his doctor and got the results of his tests. We just couldn't believe that he was declared free from cancer. Further, the unbearable pain in his leg had greatly subsided, and it has not increased since then. This incident has totally fascinated me and now my interest in pranic healing is endless.

By Marcus Ubl, Partner of Entrevo, UK.

This book is a must read for anyone that is interested in understanding not only how the body works, but how health is attained.

The author makes an eloquent distinction between 'curing' the symptoms of an ailment (allopathic medicine) and regaining health. The former doesn't treat/know the underlying health issue that the symptom springs from, whereas the latter addresses the body as a complex system and seeks to understand the factors weakening the body's defences and how to reclaim your health. You're not 'fighting' the disease, you are merely getting the body back into health and the disease condition is no longer present in the healthy state.

This is the first book I recommend to friends if they're experiencing health issues and open to new ideas. Read this book, no doubt you'll come back on here as I did and buy a few extra copies to pass on to friends/family.

Preface

By the Author

Introduction

Your health is primarily your concern, and not the physician's concern. The medical care system is only there to help you to restore and maintain your health. However, in modern times the conventional medical care system has become exceedingly expensive, highly technical, very specialized and unnecessarily complicated. It depends entirely upon intricate tests, expensive high-tech machines, powerful drugs and surgical intervention. As a result the lay person, the receiver of healthcare, can hardly be expected to help himself or his dear ones in health matters.

This problem is further compounded by newer discoveries that are made by researchers every day. They continuously put forward numerous hypotheses and theories that not only confuse the laymen, they also tell the public that the subject of health is beyond their comprehension or reach. This is how the modern healthcare system chooses to project itself to the people.

On the other hand there are many simple functional disorders like allergies, the common cold, bad breath, irritable bowels, constipation, backaches, eczemas, dandruff, etc. that medical science hopelessly fails to heal. They only manage to suppress some troublesome symptoms, but they are unable to provide lasting relief. Whereas some discoveries of modern medical science (as in surgery) are admirable, there are too many reasons to be dissatisfied with the advances in drug therapy. Today the people not only fear the costs and complications of the allopathic approach to health care, but there is a growing feeling that there are flaws in the modern medical science's approach to healing. For such reasons, in spite of the enormous research in the field of modern medicine, there is a growing interest in the simple alternatives offered by alternative holistic therapies.

In this book you learn the concept of holistic healing based on the foundations of naturopathy, water therapy and pranic healing. The recommendations made here are without any commercial considerations. The only purpose is to EMPOWER YOU, the consumer of healthcare, with insights into natural healing, healthy lifestyles and self-healing techniques. The focus is not only on treating bodily ailments, but also on treating psychological and psychosomatic disorders.

To benefit from the holistic approach to healing, you have to learn to think differently in matters of health (different from how you have been conditioned to think). Instead of looking for specific remedies for specific disorders, you have to think more basically and try to recognise the causes underlying the disorder in the body. Your approach in natural healing should not be to suppress the symptoms of an ailment, but to correct the cause and assist the natural intelligence of the body in its effort to heal itself.

The philosophy and practices taught in this book will show you how you can restore your health without depending on medicines or the medical profession. The philosophy is simple to understand and the practices are easy to use. Further, the results are self-evident. So they do not need much convincing or complicated proving. In many cases, to overcome the cause of illnesses in your body you may have to only change some of your eating habits!

The natural healing systems regard *Toxaemia* to be the underlying cause of ailments in the body. Toxaemia is simply the condition of a 'diseased state' that arises due to the accumulation of toxins in the body at the cellular level. The deeper causes of Toxaemia may be due to the lifestyle or psychological factors.

Hence, an ailment in the body is considered as an effect at the functional and structural level of causes that lie inside the person; the body is like the soil in which a disease has taken root; and the treatment is directed to restore the imbalance that has arisen in the body at the many levels. Once some balance is restored, the natural intelligence of the body will take over and do the healing.

How does 'healing' differ from the notion of 'curing'?

Orthodox medical science thinks of a disease in terms of infections and chemical deficiency. Hence, they consider a disease in the body to be an *'outside-in'* process — a result of invasion by outside agents like germs, bacteria, viruses or parasites, or the result of a deficiency of some chemicals that have to be supplied from the outside. We have used the term 'curing' when the treatment is made to rely on external processes to restore the health.

Natural or holistic healing, on the other hand, thinks that the primary cause of the disease lies inside the person. Hence, they consider a disease in the body to be an *'inside-out'* process. The inner cause makes the person SUSCEPTIBLE to external agents of disease, like bacteria, or they generate deficiency related disorders. The inner cause is considered to be more important since it PRECEDES the external factors.

For this reason the holistic treatment focuses on correcting the 'internal causes' of the ailment. Once the internal causes are corrected, the healer has to only assist the natural intelligence of the body and allow it to do the healing. We have used the term 'healing' when the treatment is given only to facilitate the process of natural healing in the body.

The basic premise of Holistic Healing

When you think holistically, you do not consider your health to depend on external factors like medicines or the medical profession. Instead you will hold that it depends more on how you conduct yourself – your diet, habits, lifestyle and psychology.

You don't have to know the nature of diseases or the functions of the body parts in detail to be able to use holistic methods to heal yourself. You have to only think in terms of the imbalance in the body and assist the natural intelligence of the body in its effort to do the healing.

Thus, you can learn to maintain your health by your own efforts and, except in extreme cases, you won't need to refer to doctors. This know-how is adequately provided in this book. Your success, however, will depend on clearly you understand the principles and on how well you implement these methods.

The 'alternative therapies' discussed in this book follow the holistic approach to health. Hence, they are more like 'a way'. You have to apply the techniques WITHIN the context of the holistic philosophy and not as isolated cures.

Further, when you use holistic methods, do not look upon the body as a machine or a biological system. Instead consider it as something that is sensitive to the inner life – to your thoughts, emotions, attitudes and the life-force itself. Further, your aim is always to restore the health not to cure the disease (which usually means relieving some symptoms). For example, when you think holistically you don't think of curing asthma, but you'll think in terms of healing the person who has asthma!

A personal note

Over the past fifty years conventional medical research has been largely driven by the commercial interests of the pharmaceutical companies and other beneficiaries of the drug industry. For this reason it is not unusual to find many of their findings to be 'made to order'. Many findings are only suggestive, but they are passed on as facts that are then used to generate business profits. There is sufficient reason to be suspicious of recommendations made on the basis of statistics and random researches. They may not be worthless, but they can be very misleading. Hence, in this book we have chosen to rely on solutions that are derived from time-tested principles. We are not easily swayed by the words 'new', 'modern', 'latest', etc.

Both the principles of holistic healing and the corrective measures that are used to restore health are discussed here. Although the corrective measures or remedies are written by us, they have been around in some form or other for centuries. What is recommended here is time-tested and sufficiently tried out. However, is still up to you to get these remedies to work for you. And in this task you may not receive much help from the conventional medical practitioner. The modern physician is 'licensed' and therefore obliged to follow the 'established protocol' of the modern medical science; and some of the recommendations made in this book can amount to 'unacceptable procedures' for them.

An Overview of the Chapters

- The 'Forward' and 'Preface' tell you the point of view adopted in this book.

- Chapter-1 discusses the basic concept of holistic healing.

- Chapter-2 explains the rationale of naturopathy.

- Chapter-3 discusses the most convenient and effective remedies for self-healing.

- Chapter-4 explores the deeper causes, like stress, trauma, psychosomatic and emotional disorders, and karma. These causes underlie the basic disease factor of Toxaemia in the body.

- Chapter-5 discusses the theory and practice of pranic healing, which is exceptionally useful in healing deeper organ troubles, backaches, psychosomatic disorders and psychological troubles.

Acknowledgements

This book started out in 2006 as a small booklet titled *Health & Healing without Drugs*. It was based on some insights I acquired from Dr. Sukhbir Singh, a senior naturopath. My wife, Kalpana, helped me very much in formulating some of the concepts contained in that book. Later in that year, based on that book, I conducted a half-day program on *Natural & Holistic Healing* for the group, *'Women in Government',* in New York. Subsequently, in 2008, 2011, 2013, and 2017 Madanda Machayya organised repeat health workshops in USA. I've taken these opportunities to improve the presentation and make it more complete. The chapters on Pranic Healing, Emotional Causes of health disorders, etc. have been freshly re-written.

I wish to thank the participants of my workshops and many friends who have encouraged me to put together my findings in this book for the benefit of the ailing public. In particular, I'm grateful to Dr. Frank Sanchez and Dr. Madanda Machayya for writing the FOREWORD; and to my daughter, Aarti, for making the SKETCHES for the chapter on Pranic Healing. I also thank the readers for contributing their book REVIEWS.

Chapter-1:

Holistic Healing

1. What are the limitations of allopathic treatment?

The Medicine Show (A Consumer Union of U.S. Publication) says: *"The public has grown accustomed to thinking that a doctor's job in curing diseases is to find the cause and remove it. However, the truth is that a greater part of the physician's efforts goes towards relieving symptoms with very little knowledge of their causes; and today's most prevalent illnesses, many of which are chronic illnesses, are merely treated symptomatically."*

ALLOPATHIC (modern) medicine is the mainstream system. It is a leader for treatment in emergencies, in infectious diseases and in ailments that require surgical intervention. However, most of the common troubles that people face are FUNCTIONAL DISORDERS, such as: *respiratory disorders* like allergies, colds, coughs; *skin disorders* like eczema, itching, dandruff, psoriasis, foul odour; *pains* like headache, stiff-joints, back pains; *digestive disorders* like irritable bowels, constipation, flatulence, etc.

For such troubles, the allopathic medical system provides no effective remedy. It only tries to manage or relieve some symptoms of the disorder. In this way it provides some temporary relief.

2. What is so wrong with relieving symptoms?

All medicines modify some symptoms, particularly the irritating ones. During the time of treatment the body will, on its own, heal itself. However, if the underlying disease factor remains unattended, the treatment gives an 'illusion of cure'. Newer symptoms will keep on cropping up from time to time!

Drug therapy is useful in treating acute diseases, particularly when the symptoms are severe or life threatening. However, when you habitually treat symptoms with drugs, the symptoms themselves get modified and develop chronic disorders like headaches, stuffed nose, acidity, wheezing, rheumatism, eczema, allergy, blood pressure, etc. These disorders are less intense in their effect, but they harass more since they last longer and recur periodically!

For such chronic disorders there are *'no outright cures'* – there are only medications that can temporally manage or relieve the symptoms. The patient is put on medication that has to be taken for the rest of their life! Thus, the patient is never healed. Treatment is only directed to controlling some irritating symptoms.

This trend has become set in modern times due to the commercial interests of the healthcare business. The companies are mainly interested in developing highly profitable solutions that require long term use of drugs or surgical intervention. Hence, hypertension is not healed; it is treated with BP pills that have to be taken for a lifetime. Asthma is not healed; inhalers are constant companions of the afflicted. Osteoarthritis is not healed; the ultimate remedy is sought in knee replacement. Allergies are not healed; the victim becomes increasingly dependent on medication. The list is endless.

Further, when the patient continues to use a medicine, the response to the medicine diminishes. However, that does not trouble the advocates of the drug therapy. Instead, the pharmaceutical companies keep on rejuvenating their business by creating a demand for the newer drugs and procedures that are poured into the market every day. The patient is made to think that someday 'scientific research' will develop a cure for their disease. However, that day is not going to come. They would do much better if they begin to look for their remedy elsewhere.

The central problem of modern medicine (the drug therapy and surgical intervention) in treating diseases is that they deal with the END of the disease spectrum and concentrate only on its localised manifestation. But most of the disease processes in the early stages are merely functional disorders. The modern medical science chooses to ignore their causes and uses the drug therapy to suppress the symptoms of the acute disorder. In this way they allow the diseased state to develop further. They assume that their task is to deliver immediate results by merely suppressing the symptoms! But when the cause is allowed to continue, the diseased state gets internalised and gradually the body structures and organs start to break down. That does not seem to bother the medical industry, because now they demonstrate their expensive wonders of surgery.

Modern medical science has misrepresented the true nature of a disease by considering it as merely the effect on the physical body, which can be removed by external means like drugs and surgery. Hence, the attention of the people has been distracted from knowing the true cause of their disease, and from looking in the right places for the true remedy.

We repeat: Symptoms are not the disease. They are only the results of the disorder. The true cause of disease always lies inside the person — in their mindset, lifestyle and emotions. Hence, if you do not correct the causes inside the person, you do not really attempt to heal.

3. What is the difference between a holistic approach and a specialised approach?

When symptoms are seen in the context of the whole person, they take on a totally different significance than when they are seen in the context of an ailing part of the body. When you think analytically, you simply REDUCE the level of the insight from the whole to the part. Then you only see the disorder in the parts and the symptoms. And as a result your treatment will be directed to relieving the symptoms or surgically cutting up the part.

However, when the underlying cause is elsewhere in the system (as in the eating habit), then you can miss it completely. This is precisely what happens when the health problem arises due to a disorder in the functioning of the whole person, as in psychosomatic disorders or a faulty eating habit. The disorder simply shows itself as symptoms in the parts. In such a case if the treatment is aimed at merely curing the part, then it can only provide some temporary relief. The underlying 'disease factor' will continue, and so the symptoms will play hide and seek.

From the holistic point of view, the solutions that emerge from a fragmented perspective themselves become problems for the whole! They give some temporary relief to the part, but they create bigger long-term problems for the whole. The disorder cannot be truly irradiated without correcting the cause in the whole.

Further, the quick fix cures that are used disturb the natural feedback system the body uses to heal itself. Then the natural healing processes get obstructed, and you have to depend more on external measures to give relief. In this context it is significant to note the observation of a 15th century physician, PARACELSUS: *The disease does not change its state to accommodate itself to the knowledge of the physician; it is for the physician to arrive at an understanding of the true causes of the disease.*

4. What is holistic about healing?

The holistic therapies do not focus on merely relieving symptoms. Instead, they try to perceive the underlying CAUSE of the ailment, which more often in the whole person; that is in his or her habits and tendencies. The saying is: *"You are not ill or diseased in a part. The symptoms of the disease are expressed in a part, or it is the 'weakest link' in the body that has broken down."*

When health problems are considered in this way, your aim to correct the cause in the 'whole person' and not merely treat the symptoms of a 'disease syndrome'. Thus, in addition to treating a particular disorder in a body part, the errors in the lifestyle and habits are also corrected.

Most of the holistic therapies have a simplistic diagnosis for the most complex physical disorders. For example, Ayurveda will talk in terms of 'Tridosha'; Naturopath will talk in terms of 'Toxaemia'; Water Cure will talk in terms of 'Dehydration', Psychic Healing will talk in terms of 'Prana Deficiency', Homoeopathy will talk in terms of 'Constitutional Remedy', etc. However, the simplicity in diagnosis should not be mistaken for a lack of sophistication or effectiveness. The remedies they provide are not only effective, but often their effectiveness is amazing.

If someone is looking here for a one to one correspondence between a disease and a remedy, they are unlikely to find it. For example, the holistic systems cannot have a cure for baldness, asthma or diabetes. These therapies do not work like that. They look upon the symptoms of a disease as merely a result of disorder in the body. Their focus is on correcting the cause of the disorder. When the cause is corrected, the disease more often loses its grip on the patient. Then the natural intelligence of the body will take over and do the healing. If some symptoms still remain, they will respond to almost any kind of therapy.

Although the modern super-specialised physicians talk of diseases in very complex terms, the 'complexity' around the disorder is something that is created by them. It has arisen due to the way in which the modern medical science has chosen to evolve its solutions or cures. However, it does not make them superior. Instead there are greater benefits to be had by looking at your health problems differently. If you examine the results of the alternative therapies with an open mind, you will find a great consistency in the healing.

5. Is there a change in the concept of responsibility?

People enter the holistic field through the doors of 'curiosity' or 'crisis'. They just want to know something different; they want to try out alternatives; or they are desperate because the orthodox medical treatment has left them hopeless. In either case they are reaching out to a *'different approach'* to health and healing.

Although the patients are willing to try out new approaches, they still come to the healer with an 'orthodox mindset'. That is, they expect to remain passive and want the healer will do all the curing! They fail to understand that the role of the healer in the holistic approach is to only facilitate the healing process and not to provide an external cure. The responsibility always rests with the patient. The patient will get the assistance they need, but they cannot abdicate their responsibility of health to the healer.

Further, as the treatment continues, sooner or later the patient will come face to face with the very aspect of their life that they have been trying to avoid confronting. From the holistic point of view, to allow them to avoid facing it would be to allow the source of the illness to continue! So the healers can become insistent and some patients become uncomfortable and drop out.

In the initial phase the treatment usually focuses on relieving the toxaemia or the primary disease factor in the body. But in the next phase the focus will be on making the necessary changes in the lifestyle habits and emotions that had generated the toxaemia. The patients can only be explained what needs to be changed, but they have to make the changes for themselves. Nobody can do it for them. The patient has to cultivate faith in the holistic philosophy to really benefit from it.

The role of the patient in holistic therapy is that of an active 'participant'. He or she cannot remain a passive recipient of the treatment.

Chapter-2:

Naturopathy

A. *Healing in terms of the vital force*

1. What is the cause of disease in the body?

Whenever there is a physical or emotional disturbance in our life, the vital force in the body gets depleted. The physical disturbance can be due to prolonged tension, upset digestion or some emotional disturbance like trauma or excessive change.

However, once the vital force is depleted, it becomes insufficient. Then the normal functions of the body get disturbed. The process ultimately results in the accumulation of toxins or waste products in the body. This accumulation reduces the body's resistance to the external agents of disease like allergens, germs, etc. and makes it SUSCEPTIBLE to illness.

Here we provide a simple understanding of how the body works in terms of 'toxaemia' and 'vital force'.

2. What is the vital force and what functions does it perform in our body?

Our body remains alive and functions as a whole due to the presence of a vital force or prana in it. The vital force is something subtle, like electricity. It animates the whole body and flows as currents along the nerves and vital channels of the body. Thereby it keeps the body working as a whole.

When the vital force is *abundant* and it flows smoothly, the body functions properly. Then we feel light and alert. When this force becomes *weak* or its flow through the vital channels is disturbed, the functions of the body get disturbed. Then we experience fatigue, sluggishness, and an upset feeling; or we become restless and irritable.

The vital force performs the functions of digestion, assimilation and elimination in the body. Through *digestion* it transforms the food into material that the body can use. Through *assimilation* it transforms the digested food into body tissue or oxidises it to generate energy. And through *elimination* it removes the waste products. That is, it decomposes the waste, poisonous and dead materials so that they can be easily eliminated from the body.

Thus, digestion and assimilation are said to be the health building functions, whereas elimination is said to be the cleansing and repairing function. All these functions are complementary and the body performs them simultaneously or side by side.

3. What exactly happens when the vital force becomes weak?

Once the body's vital force becomes weak, our digestion, assimilation and elimination also become weak. Then our system becomes sluggish, our digestion is incomplete, our assimilation is poor, and all this undigested and unassimilated stuff has to be decomposed and thrown out. The elimination is also sluggish and so there is a gradual build up of toxins in the body. When the toxin level is more that the body can tolerate, the condition is called TOXAEMIA.

Once there is Toxaemia in the body, the work of elimination becomes most crucial factor for our health. It becomes the bottleneck health issue. Then the natural intelligence of the body will focus most of its energy on eliminating the accumulated toxins from the body.

At such times, it is necessary to *conserve* our energy so that the body can perform the extra work of cleaning effectively. ***The natural instinct of the body is to rest and abstain from eating***. If we eat at such times, the food remains undigested and becomes an extra load on our system. Instead, if we take rest and abstain from eating, the natural intelligence of the body and the body organs will use their 'reserve vital force' to cleanse our system from 'inside out'.

Thus, the cleansing function begins automatically in the body when we provide the condition of 'total rest' – rest from both digestion and physical effort.

4. Why does the vital force become weak?

The vital force is INHERENT in all living systems. It sustains the body functions and also performs the function of healing. This force becomes weak or dysfunctional when we eat too much or eat food that is hard to digest, when we continuously take drugs or stimulants, when we indulge in excessive sex, when we take insufficient sleep or rest, or when there is dehydration in the body.

Further, the vital force is very sensitive to our emotions and feelings. Hence, the vital force becomes weak when we are emotionally disturbed (due to fear, anger or sadness); when we lose hope; when we act against our conscience (break the moral law); or when there is excessive change in our life (divorce, change of job, residence, etc.). Besides these reasons the vital force also declines naturally with age.

5. How can we restore the vital force?

Once the vital force has become weak, the quickest way to restore it is by fasting, resting, drinking fresh water, nurturing positive feelings, etc. FAITH is a big rejuvenator of the vital force. However, faith in a doctor or medicine is a poor substitute for direct faith in the natural law or a benevolent higher power.

Some people mistake the vital force for MUSCULAR ENERGY. However, the vital force is something that animates the body the body organs and the body cells. It circulates as currents in the entire body and thereby maintains all the body functions. Hence, restoring the vital force is more like overcoming the fatigue of the nervous system.

The body can also rejuvenate its vital force by drawing it (prana) from external sources like food, air, earth, sunlight and water. It can also be drawn from other people and the healer. However, essentially the vital force is something that arises from within the body, from inside the body organs and cells. Sleep also rejuvinates the vital force.

B. Some issues of Natural Healing

1. What is the central idea of natural healing?

Once waste and toxins have accumulated in the body, the body processes will try to expel them. The process of eliminating the toxins from the body gives rise to a numerous symptoms of the mind and body. However, these functional and pathological symptoms arise as a part of the body's effort to expel the accumulated toxins. Hence, they should be considered as by-products of the healing process. They are a part of the natural purification process that is referred to as an 'elimination crises' in naturopathy.

So, if we apply curative measures, it should not be to suppress the normal response of the body. It should be to remove the cause of the illness. That is, we should assist the cleansing effort of the body and not obstruct it by suppressing the symptoms!

2. What happens when we suppress the symptoms with drugs?

The body works like a system in which the different functions are regulated through a natural *feedback* mechanism. Feedback means that the body is using the result or effect that arises to guide its next action.

Example, when there is less water in the body we get the sensation of thirst; and we satiate the thirst by drinking more water. Hence, the sensation of thirst is necessary to make us drink the extra water we need. In other words, the symptoms of an illness provide the body with the information it needs to perform the task of healing or repair effectively.

For example, let us consider the symptom of FEVER. The body increases its temperature to help the white blood cells fight and overcome the increased concentration of bacteria. However, if we suppress the symptom of fever with drugs like Aspirin or Paracetamol, then we have to use still more 'external agents' like antibiotics to destroy the excess bacteria, since at lowered temperature the white blood cannot do its job effectively.

Thus, whenever we suppress body symptoms artificially with drugs, we disturb the *'natural feedback mechanism'* that our body uses to carry out the cleansing and repair work! As a result the body is unable to perform its self-healing function, and the cleansing action has also to be stimulated artificially, with more drugs. And these drugs themselves increase the toxic load in the body. The end result is that the body's natural ability to heal itself is progressively lost!

Let us see what happens when we are careless in our eating habits. Then we may eat too much sweets or fried food. *What happens?* At first the digestion gets disturbed. Then the food is not completely digested. The undigested food is difficult to assimilate. Hence, there is an increase in the food products that have to be decomposed and eliminated from the body.

This results in an excess load on decomposition. Some food products remain partly decomposed; and these incompletely decomposed waste products irritate the mucus membrane and increase the expectoration. So there is an excess of discharges. We can suppress these discharges with anti-histamines, but if the build-up of toxins continues we can develop coughs and catarrhs.

So, whenever we suppress the symptoms, the toxaemia usually increases and the disease progresses inward – from the outer organs into the inner more vital organs like the lungs and liver. Then the lungs can develop the symptoms of bronchial asthma. Again, we can relieve the symptoms by using dilators (chemicals) to ease the breathing. However, all these drugs only increase the toxin level in the organs and make them more susceptible to infection. Then, ultimately we can develop bigger disorders like pneumonia or a patch in the lungs.

3. Aren't germs and bacteria the causes of disease?

Modern medical science has made us believe that germs, bacteria, microbes, viruses and parasites are the causes of our diseases. However, naturopathy considers them to be only the *external agents* of the disease and not the internal causes. Just as flies breed where we keep garbage, so also germs breed easily when the body or an organ is loaded with toxins!

Germs and bacteria are merely nature's scavengers that mainly carry out the function of decomposing or fermenting the dead material in the body. They are harmless against healthy living cells. *Hence, the germs become a complicating factor in a disease only AFTER the conditions of disease, the toxaemia, already exists.* Once waste matter accumulates and the cells lose their vitality, the bacteria can decompose them and feed on them. However, in the healthy condition the cells are not affected by bacteria. Further, the by-products of bacterial decomposition become dangerous only when they accumulate. So, as long as our body is able to eliminate these toxins, there is nothing to fear from germs and bacteria!

Thus, we should regard an infection as a subsequent complication that arises when the primary cause of illness, the toxaemia, already exists. We should not consider the disease as an attack by germs. The germs only grow when the body or body organ has become vulnerable. And if that is true, it is more appropriate to focus on building your immunity and resistance to germs and bacteria by detoxifying your system than to focus on destroying all the external agents of disease.

4. What is the natural self-healing principle?

According to naturopathy *healing is a biological process, and the affected organism has in it the power to heal itself.* Then what do the drugs do? Drugs can stimulate the vital force to do the healing, but by themselves the drugs cannot heal.

Every living organism has an inherent capacity to heal itself. That is to say it has a vital force that has a regenerative capacity that is capable of restoring its healthy functioning. However, once the vital force becomes weak, the body is unable to conduct its vital functions properly. Then undigested materials and metabolic wastes accumulate in the tissues and cells of the body and ultimately give rise to the condition of toxaemia. This 'diseased condition' is experienced as irritation, uneasiness, weakness and restlessness.

Once toxaemia exists, sooner or later the body will try to expel the toxins. The elimination effort, with or without complications from the disease agents like germs, will give rise to many symptoms in the mind and body such as fevers, catarrhs, inflammations, headaches, phobias, etc. All such symptoms, except where degeneration of organs is involved, are signs of toxaemia. Toxaemia simply means that the body has more toxins than it can tolerate in its present state of vitality.

The natural remedy in all such cases is to provide complete rest. The body always has a reserve of vital force, and when we provide the condition of 'total rest', the natural intelligence of the body will use its reserve vital force to do the most important work of removing the toxins. Once the toxin level in the body is reduced, the vital force will once again begin to function normally. Then the symptoms of the illness will naturally begin to disappear.

5. Which organs of the body perform the elimination function?

The body normally eliminates waste through the bowels, kidneys, lungs and skin. It is discharged as stools, urine, breath, and sweat respectively. In addition to these, there are other organs that have a special connection with the function of elimination. They are the LIVER, the SPLEEN and the MUCOUS MEMBRANE.

The liver breaks down toxic chemicals and drugs from the blood stream. The spleen destroys bacteria, viruses and weak cells from the blood and lymphatic system and is a part of the body's immune system. And the mucous membranes remove the toxins from the lymphatic system through mucous discharges.

6. Do laxatives reduce Toxaemia?

The elimination that is sought by the natural healing systems is the work of removing the toxins from the cells and tissues of the body. It is not merely the waste from the bowels. It is called 'internal cleansing', and it should not be confused with the limited cleansing or evacuation that is performed by laxatives and enemas!

Further, the limited cleansing that is brought about by laxatives is done by irritating the intestines. Hence, they increase the burden on the body and there are better ways to do this.

7. Why is the direction of natural healing said to be *'inside out'*?

The natural process of healing happens by throwing the dead tissue and waste products out of the body. For example, a *bilious headache* disappears when the toxins in the stomach are eliminated. (Such things happen in a system because the seemingly 'isolated parts' of the system are actually inter-connected). Aspirin can only temporarily remove the sensation of this headache, whereas the internal cleansing (induced by drinking salt water) will remove both the sensation and the bilious congestion. In the same way *ointments* can be used to hold moisture on the skin and suppress the symptoms of dryness or rash, whereas the internal cleansing will naturally hydrate the skin and keep it glowing.

The natural DIRECTION OF HEALING in the body is an 'inside-out' process. That is the body will remove the toxins from the inner, more vital organs onto the outer, less vital organs, and if the process is allowed to continue, the toxins will be eliminated from the body. However, if this normal direction of cure is obstructed or altered, the toxins can move inward to the more vital, internal organs and into the nerves and mind. Then, the disease is said to progress inward, where it becomes more dangerous.

The symptom of ECZEMA arises on the skin when the skin is trying to relieve the toxic load in the body. If you suppress this condition with ointments, the symptoms may shift onto the *lungs*. Then the lungs will try to remove the toxins through their secretions. However, these secretions can become sticky and cause difficulty in breathing at night. So, you may relieve the condition with expectorants and dilators. But these drugs also contribute their share of toxins to the body. So ultimately an elimination crisis will arise.

However, if you assist the body in eliminating the toxins, first the breathing trouble will disappear and the itching will resurface on the skin. If you remover the internal causes, the discharges will gradually reduce the toxin level, and ultimately the eczema will simply disappear.

In the same way, when a CATARRH develops in the nose, you should consider it as a sign that tells you to facilitate the cleansing. Instead, if you choose to suppress the discharges with nasal drops, the load falls on an internal organ, such as the liver, which becomes sluggish. However, if you increase the internal cleansing, it will relieve both the liver trouble and the catarrh.

8. Do medicines cure the disease?

The people have the belief that medicines actually cure diseases. However, this is a deception. Medicines, drugs and vaccines do not play a direct part in the cure. That is to say, *the medicines do not create new cells or repair damaged tissue. It is the natural self-healing power within the body and the body organs that actually cures and restores their healthy functioning.* The medicines only have the power to alter the symptoms of a disease!

Then why do we take medicines? The medicines have to power to alter the symptoms around and make them manageable. And during that time the natural intelligence of the body performs the healing. However, if the cause is allowed to remain, the diseased state will continue and sooner or later the symptoms will recur or newer symptoms will arise.

What is the function of medicines in healing? In holistic treatment the function of medicines, if any, is similar to the function of a doctor in fixing a broken bone. The doctor's task is to align the bone pieces and keep them held together in a plaster so that the vital force can do the repair. In the same way the doctor can create the conditions that help or support the natural healing process. Medicines can be used to serve a similar function. However, when we use medicines, we have to take care that they *create the conditions that assist the natural self-healing processes in the body and do not create complications, side-effects and after-effects.*

9. What is the effect of drugs on the body?

The primary effect of drugs is on the symptoms in the body. They can relieve some annoying symptoms and provide some temporary relief. And during that time the reserve vital force may restore the body functions.

However, there are some drugs, like the ANTIBIOTICS, act directly on the disease agents or bacteria in the body and destroy them. However, they also destroy the useful bacteria and generate another kind of imbalance in the body. Further, these drugs are not nutrients. They are more like poisonous intrusions into the body that work in an artificial way. All of them have side-effects and after-effects, which cause many other disturbances in the body. Some of these disturbances are known, but there can be many more disturbances that will arise in time which are not clearly understood. Hence, using this kind of drug therapy cannot be the preferred way to go about doing things, particularly when there are viable alternatives.

Further, by removing the bacteria or the disease propagating agent, as in the antibiotic therapy, we have still not restored health. If the underlying condition of toxaemia is not relieved, the person is still susceptible to other disease propagating agents. For this reason any remedial measure that is directed at relieving only some disease factors, WITHOUT removing the toxaemia is usually only a partial solution.

HOMEOPATHS also believe that the symptoms of an illness arise in the body due to the malfunctioning of the vital force. Hence, they do not suppress the symptoms. Instead, they use the 'totality of symptoms' to find a 'constitutional remedy' for the patient. This remedy acts directly on the vital force and stimulates it to carry out the work of eliminating the toxins from inside out. However, the eating habits, the lifestyle and the emotional disturbances remain unattended in the Homeopathic treatment. Hence, there will again be a toxin build up in the body. So the patient will keep on returning to the doctor for assistance, and this returning can continue for a lifetime!

In the method of 'pranic healing' also, the healer removes the congestion in the flow of vital force in the body. This creates a sudden burst of vitality. It has the effect of detoxifying the organs and it can directly relieve many annoying symptoms. Again, if such a treatment is not followed up by attending to the deeper causes, the diseased condition will tend to recur!

10. Are there dangers in using drug therapy?

All the parts of the human system are interrelated. Therefore, when we manipulate the symptoms in one part of the body without attending to the underlying disease factor, newer symptoms will arise naturally in another part. Hence, every drug induces some disturbance inside the body, which can be called its 'secondary disease'. For this reason all drugs have SIDE EFFECTS. Some of these side effects appear immediately, and some of them pass through many stages and show up after a long time as AFTER EFFECTS. For example, taking birth control pills may show up as a defect in the uterus in the offspring. If this factor is understood, it is evident that many chronic disorders that we come across in today's society are actually *'drug induced side effects'*.

The drugs are poisonous intrusions into the body that the body has to ultimately eliminate. So, when we continuously use drugs to manage our chronic symptoms, many complications will arise. Further, if we keep on treating our body in this way, we are preparing the ground for bigger structural disorders to arise in our vital organs! Thus, *drug treatment, instead of curing us, actually makes us susceptible to greater disorders of the vital organs like heart, liver, lungs and kidney.* For such reasons it is not safe to use the drug therapy; and drugs are dangerous to our health.

The tendency in orthodox medicine is to treat the symptoms of chronic diseases with drugs. This results in drug overuse, which is always dangerous due to the complications that arise, and due to the side-effects and after effects that catch up. So, very often after one specialist has cured a patient, we find that the patient is being treated by another specialist. In this way the treatment becomes endless and burdensome. Thus, whatever relief the drugs provide us comes at a heavy cost, and the drug therapy more often only POSTPONES our return to natural health.

11. When should we take treatment with drugs?

All kinds of treatments are legitimate in their place. Hence, there is a place for the drug therapy. It can be very useful when you are treating serious infections or acute diseases like malaria, pneumonia, typhoid, hepatitis-b, etc. In these ailments the situations develop very rapidly, and they can be life threatening or difficult to manage. Hence, you should consult a doctor who uses the drug therapy to give immediate relief.

However, you must understand that when there is acute disease or infection in the body, the condition of toxaemia already exists. The acute condition has developed because the immunity was low, and the lowered immunity was due to the accumulation of toxins in the body. Hence, immediately after the acute disease subsides, you should undertake a program for detoxification.

12. What is the difference between an acute disease and an elimination crisis?

Symptoms like giddiness, purging, vomiting, fever, inflammation, headache, catarrh, foul discharges, weakness, etc., develop when the body is throwing out the toxins from the cells and organs. Such symptoms are a part of the natural healing process and they should not be confused with the symptoms of an infection that arises in the case of an acute disease.

When the body is removing the toxins from the deeper organs or in a long standing disorder, the symptoms can become intense. Then an 'elimination crises' arises. However, such symptoms must not be treated and suppressed with drugs. These symptoms only have to be MANAGED. When the toxin level in the body is reduced, these symptoms will subside naturally.

13. Are there other food items that are as harmful as drugs?

The word 'drug' is normally used to refer to chemical substances that are commonly used as medications. However, natural healing systems use the term in a much wider sense to INCLUDE harmful substances like nicotine (tobacco), caffeine (coffee), alcohol (drinks), aspirin (pain killers), theobromine (cocoa), theophilline (tea), and refined sugar.

The habitual use of such items produces an addiction, and many side-effects. Hence, regular use of such substances should be avoided as far as possible.

14. An Overview

Our lifestyle, unnatural habits, negative emotions, etc. first weaken the *vital force*.

When the vital force has become weak, many *functional disorders* develop in the body.

When these disorders are allowed to continue or when the symptoms of a disorder are habitually suppressed with drugs, the condition of *toxaemia* (increased toxins) develops in the body.

Once there is toxaemia in the body, the reserve vital force will try to detoxify the body. And in the process many symptoms will arise, which are a part of an *elimination crisis*.

These symptoms should be managed and not suppressed with drugs.

Gradually the toxin level in the body will reduce and the body's resistance to ailments will improve and the patient begins to feel much better.

However, if the symptoms that arise in an elimination crisis are *suppressed* with drugs, they get modified and become *chronic* disorders (they last a long time or recur periodically).

Then we have to keep on managing them with medication. Hence, we become unnecessarily dependent on medication, which may have to be continued for a lifetime!

In the mean while the toxaemia will get established in our

body and make some *vital organs* dysfunctional.
Then some *structural disorders* may develop that require surgical intervention.

C. An Estimate

1. What is the message of natural healing?

The natural healing systems hold that there is only one underlying cause of diseases in the body (toxaemia), which manifests itself in different forms. Accordingly, there is just one remedy: ***Remove the accumulated toxins from the body.***

Thus, there is one primary disease factor in the body, and to overcome it there is just one remedial measure – detoxification.

However, to remove the Toxaemia many measures can be used such as fasting and rest, cleansing diets, water therapy, etc. When you heal the body in this way, you will not need to take medicines.

In the process of natural healing an 'elimination crisis' may arise. At such times you have to take total rest and use measures that assist the body in eliminating the toxins. Once the toxin level has reduced, the symptoms of illness will begin to disappear on their own.

Thus, natural healing promote '*self-healing*' and does not pretend to '*cure*'. Here, healing is not something that is done to you while you remain passive. The healing process requires your active participation. Your task is to change the habits that generate the toxaemia in your body. Then all you have to do to stay healthy is provide the body with good nutrition, good elimination and adequate vital force and the body will maintain itself.

2. If natural healing is so simple, why is it not popular?

The principles of natural healing are not new. They have been known for hundreds of years. Many natural healing therapies have existed over the centuries and they are still in use today. The results that are got through such therapies are SELF-EVIDENT. Hence, there is no need for external verification through proofs.

However, the SIMPLICITY of the message of natural healing seems to be its biggest obstacle! Educated people, particularly the sophisticated medical practitioners and the researchers, just cannot believe that healing can be so simple. Normally a physician undergoes ten years of training in orthodox medicine, whereas the people who practice holistic therapies may not have taken any formal medical education or certification.

Thus, orthodox medical practitioners are unwilling to give holistic therapy the recognition or consideration it deserves. They prefer to refer to these therapists as 'quacks' or magicians (meaning deceivers), and they proclaim that they are here to protect you from being fooled by such deceivers. In addition, the common man fears naturopathy because they confuse their message of fasting with starvation. The people imagine that the treatment will be very severe and too unsettling for their liking. Hence, they fear it and avoid it.

Perhaps the greatest obstacle to natural healing therapies is that people do not want to accept the responsibility for their health. Accepting the responsibility would require them to give up some of their habits that have become the cause of their illness. However, most people are unwilling to make the effort to change their lifestyle or eating habits. They would rather put their faith in medicines and hope something new will be discovered in time, which will cure them. Otherwise they prefer to take a pill and settle for some temporary relief, and believe it is the best they can do.

3. What kind of illnesses does natural healing cure?

Fasting, elimination diets, water therapy, etc. will overcome most of the FUNCTIONAL DISORDERS in your mind and body. They will relieve phobias, irritability, hypertension, depression, sexual disorders, stuffed nose, coughs, catarrhs, allergies, asthma, stiff joints, rheumatism, eczema, rashes, digestive disorders (diarrhoea, irritable bowels, ulcers, acidity, tooth decay, constipation and flatulence), sleeplessness, obesity, headaches, weakness of hearing, seeing or smelling, etc.

All you have to do is understand the principles of natural healing and follow a detoxification program for a few months. Then you will see the amazing results by yourself. You will *overcome your dependency* on drugs and doctors for a lifetime! However, where there is already a significant structural damage to the organs, as in cancer, emphysema, hernia, heart disease, etc., or if your ailment is due to an injury, you will have to visit the doctor.

4. Why does modern medical science search only for external cures?

Modern medical science looks for external cures for diseases due to their *'concept of disease'*. If you consider a disease as the consequence of an ATTACK upon the body by outside agents like germs, then you will seek to destroy these outside agents. This trend has generated a basic error of perception. This error has arisen from the great success that modern medicine had in dealing with epidemics in the earlier part of the last century. The trend has been set and now it continues.

It is important to note that the germs can come from anywhere, but to grow they need a body that is loaded with toxins. Hence, instead of focusing on destroying all the external agents of a disease, it is more appropriate to focus on building your immunity and resistance to the external agents by cleansing the system.

Let us understand why the modern medical science has no effective remedy for even simple troubles like colds, allergies, headaches, sleeplessness, lethargy, irritable bowels, foul odours, loss of hair, itching, constipation, etc. *Such ailments are actually the effects of toxaemia. Hence, they cannot be eradicated in isolation!* Instead, if you cleanse your body of toxins many of these irritating symptoms will disappear on their own. And the symptoms that remain will be much easier to manage.

Chapter-3:

The Prescriptions R$_x$

- Diet and eating habits
- Nutrition
- Water therapy
- Bath & Packs
- The cleansing diet
- The therapeutic fast
- A schedule for implementation

A. Diet and Eating Habits

1. What is the natural health prescription?

a) R$_x$: *'Eat less and take only easy-to-digest food.'*

When you take in just sufficient food, you do not waste your energy on processing the excess food. Further, when you digest all the food you eat, you become more energetic and produce fewer toxins.

b) When undigested food remains in the body it ferments, and that gives rise to toxins in the body. Hence, you should value the food items *according to your ability to digest* and assimilate them, and not by their nutrient content! Don't judge the value of the food from the chart given on the package. Avoid eating food that is indigestible or toxic; and that includes all kind of food that is fried, mixed with soybeans, or made from refined flour.

c) Avoid consuming food that is highly processed, highly sweetened or salted, and foods that carry health claims (don't encourage deceivers). Food is processed to increase its shelf life (not your life) and the processing makes it more indigestible in your body. Further, processed foods are usually deep-fried to make them tasty and addictive ingredients are often added to increase their consumption. It's better for the seller's business, not for your body.

d) Avoid consuming 'concentrated' food-stuff. Don't be deceived by the extra nutrient value; it will be much harder to digest. Instead, eat the food that has a lower nutritional value and which comes with a lot of roughage and fibre. The fibre and roughage make it easier for the body to process and assimilate the food. The waste products that are generated from eating such foods are easier to eliminate.

e) Avoid consuming diet supplements and micronutrients unless you have a specific deficiency. And don't believe you have the deficiency because it was suggested in the newspaper. By taking such supplements you merely serve the interests of the pharmaceutical companies and not your interest. If you have a specific deficiency, take the supplement (preferably from a natural source) only until the deficiency is overcome. Do not continue to consume it thereafter. Otherwise taking the supplements can create an unnecessary DEPENDENCY or it can generate imbalance in the body.

2. What are good eating habits?

a) The main purpose of eating is to feed the body. Hence, do not combine other purposes, like parties and thrills with the act of eating.

b) While eating, remain conscious of what you are eating. When you maintain this discipline, the natural instinct of the body will awaken and you will be able to sense the quality of the food you eat and know how much is enough.

c) The stomach cannot digest the food properly when it is fully loaded. Hence, stop eating when the stomach is three-forth full.

d) Establish an eating routine and adhere to it. Don't eat between meals. If you eat at odd times, you will not be hungry at the meal time. Further, if you are not hungry at the meal time, don't feel obliged to eat. As a rule, if you are not hungry, don't eat.

e) Consume a glass of water or drinks with meals. The food will mix better and become easier to digest. However, often when we drink water during meals, we tend to wash down the food without chewing it properly. Then the food is not digested properly. Hence, avoid this habit.

f) Try to drink 'fresh stream' water and avoid drinking tap water or recycled water as far as possible.

h) The morning time is naturally suited to the function of elimination. You can assist the elimination processes at this time by doing some exercise like walking, and by drinking plenty of water.

The digestion is strongest around mid-day. Hence, the lunch should be the main meal. At other times in the day, eat little and only easy-to-digest food. The digestive fire becomes weak on overcast days and in the rainy season. Hence, eat less on such days and in the corresponding season.

3. What is the correct way of eating fruits?

Fruits can be used to detoxify the body. However, it is better to eat them on an empty stomach and not along with the meals.

What happens when you mix food with fruits?

Most fruits do not require much digestion. Hence, when fruits are eaten on an empty stomach, they are processed quickly in the stomach. However, when you eat fruits along with food that requires a lot of digestion, the fruit material stays for a long time in the stomach. Then it ferments and becomes 'acid forming'. Then the cleansing value of the fruit is lost.

Fruits, like oranges, apples and lemons may be acidic on the outside, but inside the body they have an *alkaline effect*. However, this alkaline effect happens only when the fruit is eaten in the correct way – without mixing it with other foods. Preserved fruit juices and overripe fruit usually have an acidic effect.

4. What is a natural health diet?

A sample diet:

BREAKFAST: Consume only fresh fruits or dry fruits.

LUNCH: Begin with salads and use lemon and olive oil as salad dressing. The main serving should consist of rice and lentils; or cooked vegetables and whole grain bread or chapatti. You can add eggs, cheese, yams and potatoes for variety. In addition, you can add or apply ghee (cracked butter) to the food.

SNACKS: If you must take a snack, take a beverage with two biscuits.

DINNER: Consume vegetable or lentil soup, baked or cooked vegetables along with toast or toasted chapattis (khakhra) or baked potatoes. Eat less than hunger.

5. How to adjust your diet to your health condition

Here are some practical suggestions for adjusting your diet to suit your constitution:

When you are prone to excessive MUCOUS discharges, as in colds, catarrhs, etc. avoid eating fatty food, milk products and sweets. Instead, use of ghee, honey, salt and hot drinks. Avoid drinking cold water. It slows down the digestion. This kind of imbalance causes laziness and poor digestion.

When you experience a HOT FEELING or biliousness, avoid eating sour and unripe fruits, yoghurt, salt, cheese, hot spices (like garlic, fenugreek and mustard). Make a liberal use of leafy green vegetables, soaked nuts, sweet fruit, cumin seeds, cardamom and lentils in your diet. This kind of imbalance causes fevers, headaches, pains, loose motions and irritation.

When you experience excessive GAS problems, avoid eating melons, beans, cabbage and other gas producing food. Also, avoid taking cold or stale food. Make liberal use of vegetables, soaked nuts, sweet and sour fruits, ghee and well-toasted bread. This kind of imbalance causes insomnia, constipation, worry and mental instability.

B. Nutrition

1. What is a balanced diet?

The authors of different natural health books suggest different kinds of natural health food diets. There are so many recommendations that people find it difficult to decide what is right for them. To simplify the confusion we have explained our recommendations below.

The prescription given here is suited to persons who are in the 'fifty plus' age group. It is for people who do not do hard manual labour; who do deskwork; and who live a comfortable lifestyle under moderate climatic conditions. You can make adjustments to these recommendations according to your age, occupation, climate, and individual characteristics.

Categories	Ideal %	What people usually consume %
Fat	15	25
Protein	10	25
Carbohydrate	70	35
Sugar	5	15

The chart given above explains what would amount to a 'balanced diet'. It is a general criterion that you can use to make adjustments to your diet. For example, if you want to reduce the fat and protein in your diet, you should consume less meats, cheese, dairy products, eggs and peanut butter. If you want to increase the carbohydrate content of your diet, you should increase your intake of cereals, sweet potato, breads, etc. If you are underweight, you can consider increasing your protein intake.

Here we discuss some additional considerations for different categories of food.

2. Carbohydrates

There are different types of carbohydrates. Glucose is a sugar, which is one molecule long, whereas complex carbohydrates are multiple glucose molecules bound together. They ultimately break down in the body into molecules of glucose.

The key difference between consuming carbohydrates and sugars is that carbohydrates take much longer to get absorbed into the blood and break down into sugars. The slow absorption and breakdown rate makes it possible for the cells to store carbohydrates and release them slowly into the blood stream. Hence, the body cells can utilise them as sugars as and when energy is required.

3. Fibre

Dietary fibres can be of two kinds, soluble and insoluble. Food fibre is insoluble – it is more like indigestible and non-decomposable plant material that passes through your digestive system. Soluble fibre on the other hand is something that dissolves in water to form a gel-like substance. It slows down the absorption of sugars into the blood stream.

Soluble fibre is found in oats, barley, rice, lentils and apples. Soluble fibre passes into the blood stream, where it also has the effect of unclogging or de-scaling the blood vessels.

Insoluble fibre gives bulk to the stools and helps in processing them through the large intestines. Most vegetables and fruits are a rich source of these fibres and minerals. They also provide the micronutrients that are necessary for maintaining healthy nerve tissue.

4. Fats

Fats have a bad reputation because they are associated with obesity. However, fats are essential to life and for keeping the nervous tissue healthy. Our brain tissue consists mainly of fat. The organs in our belly float in fat. Fats are also a good store of concentrated energy, and hence they are very useful in winter time.

Like fats, *cholesterol* is also necessary for health. It is an essential constituent of cell membranes and the building block for many hormones of the body. Doctors blame it for hardening the blood vessels, but that only happens when there is inflammation of the blood vessels. Then the cholesterol combines with the fats to form crusts, which narrow or harden the blood vessels.

Further, there are *'good fats'* and *'bad fats'*: The common saturated fats are coconut oil, hydrogenated oils, animal fat like lard and tallow, and butter. They do not decompose while frying, and hence they are used for making tasty 'fried dishes'. However, inside the body they have a sticky effect and frying makes the food is harder to digest. Further, saturated fats are easily converted into body fat. Hence, they are sometimes called 'bad fats'.

On the other hand there are monounsaturated fats which are the main constituent of nuts, olive oil and ghee. Due to the 'double bond' they are a little unstable to heating and air oxidation. They have a shorter shelf life and are unsuitable for deep frying because they decompose. However, they are suited to low temperature cooking like baking and roasting. They are not sticky in the body, and hence they are called 'good fats'. It is best to use them to pour over salads, roasted vegetables, and hot rice and for coating sweets.

There are also oils from sunflower, safflower, soybean, corn, etc. that contain a high proportion of polyunsaturated fats. For some reasons they are marketed as superior oils. Most of these oils are highly processed. It is done to increase their shelf life and not your health!

5. Protein

Protein is necessary to make body tissue and to replenish the wear and tear of the body's flesh. However, people who do not do much manual labour or exercise require little protein. Usually two eggs would be sufficient for a day's requirement of protein. The normal requirement is a half gram of protein food for every kilogram of body weight. The rest would be excess.

Excess protein cannot be stored in the body without conversion into tissue. Hence, it has to be utilised for combustion in the body or it has to be decomposed and eliminated. However, the by-products of protein combustion and decomposition are toxic. Hence, they increase toxaemia in the body. So, it is better to rely more on carbohydrates for your energy requirements. They are easily stored in the body and their waste products are much easier to eliminate.

Protein is available from nuts, meats, eggs, dairy products, lentils and wheat. However, in a vegetarian diet the protein is usually not complete (it doesn't have all the essential amino acids that are necessary to produce body tissue). Hence, vegetarians should eat NUTS (soaked overnight) or use mixed grain and lentils in combination to meet their protein requirement.

6. Sugar

Sugar is excellent for generating quick energy. However, it has become our enemy because we consume it in excess. It instantly gets into the blood stream. Some of it can be stored in the liver as glycogen. If it is in excess it has to be destroyed. Otherwise, it ferments, creates acidity and irritates the mucous membranes.

7. Dairy Milk

Dairy milk is highly rated for its supply of calcium and protein to the diet. However, milk, particularly pasteurised milk, actually adds little genuine value to the diet of an adult. A lot is already written about it these days. The milk protein is not easily digested by adults. The milk becomes like a rubbery indigestible stuff in the stomach and forms thick dense mucus in the intestines. These products clog the body's delicate mucus membranes and give rise to the symptoms of lethargy, respiratory allergies and irritable bowels.

Further, the calcium from pasteurised milk and from bones or shells is not easily absorbed by the body. The calcium got from vegetable sources like sesame seeds, almonds, oranges and leafy vegetables should be preferred. Our suggestion is that if you are suffering from respiratory allergy or colitis, give up consuming milk.

Whereas many people sing praises for pasteurized milk, here we explain some of the ILL EFFECTS OF PASTEURIZATION:

Pasteurization set out to accomplish two things – to destroy certain disease-carrying germs and prevent milk from souring. The process is to keep the milk at a temperature of 145 to 150°F for at least a ½ hour, and then reduce the temperature to below 55°F.

Whereas it is beneficial to destroy the dangerous germs, pasteurization does much more – it kills BOTH the harmful and the useful germs. Then further, when milk is subjected to high temperatures for a long time, much of its nutritional value is destroyed.

8. Acid Food

In recent years the importance of the 'acid/alkaline balance' in the body has received great importance. The general idea is that 'acidity' underlies most diseased conditions. This imbalance has become more serious in our times since most of the food items available in the market are highly processed and packaged to improve their shelf life. However, and it makes them more acidic or acid forming!

In the healthy condition our body maintains the balance by buffering the excess acids with alkaline minerals like potassium, magnesium, ammonia and calcium got from the vital organs and bones. However, when acidity becomes chronic, the buffering process creates calcium deficiency (osteoporosis), muscle wasting (foul smelling discharges). The bones provide the alkaline calcium and the muscles break down to give the alkaline ammonia. The magnesium deficiency in the muscles causes cramps and acidic colon causes excessive flatulence. Ultimately the blood becomes acidic, which becomes the ground for many chronic disorders.

To remedy this condition, avoid consuming *highly acidic food*. The acidic or acid generating foods to be avoided are processed dairy products, red meats, refined cereals, dried pulses, aerated and alcoholic drinks and coffee. In particular avoid consuming aspartame sweeteners, refined sugar, tomato ketchup, cranberries, prunes, chocolates, roasted peanuts, walnuts, cashews nuts, lard, pastas, white bread, pasteurised milk, beer and ice-cream.

Mildly acidic foods should be consumed sparingly. They are: molasses, processed fruit juices, kidney beans, corn oil, whole wheat, eggs, yogurt, buttermilk, goat's milk, whole and not-fried potato, cottage cheese and tea.

On the other side *highly alkaline foods* can sometimes (not always) be used to balance the acidic effect of other foods. Such foods are maple syrup, rice syrup, onions, green vegetables, virgin olive oil and mustard oil, papaya, mangoes, watermelon, carrots, dates, resins, lettuce, cucumber, sweet potato, beets, green beans, peas, almonds and Green tea.

Mildly alkaline foods can also be used freely. They are: honey, raw brown sugar (gur), citrus fruits, mushrooms, bananas, cherries, peaches, tomatoes, tofu, fresh corn, oils from canola, sunflower seeds and sesame seeds, sprouted seeds, mung dal, grams, brown rice, barley, chestnuts and whey.

C. Water Therapy

Detoxification of the body cells can be carried out in many ways. However, the most convenient way is by using water therapy.

In a book titled: "**Your Body's Many Cries For Water**", Dr. Fereydoon Batmanghelidj says: *You are not sick. You are thirsty in your cells. So don't treat your thirst with medication, and know that soft drinks, juices and beverages do not really quench this cellular thirst. The faulty assumption that people make is that water is a passive solvent and not an 'essential nutrient'.* This doctor holds the key factor in many ailments to be UCD or 'Unintentional Chronic Dehydration'. He explains that the body needs a certain amount of water every day for the proper functioning of its organs. No other fluid (juice, milk or beverages) can act as a substitute for water. When you take other fluids, you deceive the body by quenching the thirst, but instead of satisfying the body's need for water, these fluids act as diuretics and dehydrate the body.

When the quantity of water is insufficient, the body keeps up the supply to the vital organs, which creates a deficiency for other organs. If this condition persists, a state of chronic dehydration sets in – the organs begin to accumulate toxins and malfunction. In this way he successfully treated numerous people having complaints of asthma, rheumatism, arthritis, diabetes, BP, dyspepsia, colic pains, migraines, back pains, etc. with just water. Our aim here, however, is to use the water therapy to reduce the toxaemia in the body.

1. What is the general idea behind water therapy?

Water plays a fundamental role in health when it is drunk in sufficient quantities. It not only maintains bodily health, it also relieves many health problems like fatigue, depression, skin troubles, rheumatism, irregular blood pressure, digestive disorders, etc.

People assume they drink water when they drink large quantities of tea, coffee, soft drinks, fruit juices and alcoholic drinks. However, the hydrating effect of these drinks in the body is deceptively low. As a result, over a period of time chronic dehydration sets in even though they have been drinking a lot of fluids.

For water therapy to be effective in performing cellular cleansing you have to permanently change your water drinking habits. And to do that you must first know why water is so important to the body, what happens to the body after water enters the body, and what health conditions can be traced to chronic water deficiency. Then, in addition, you must know how to apply the therapy effectively. In the following pages we provide this valuable information.

2. What is the nature of the water content of your body?

About 70% of the body consists of water. However, the body fluids are not mixed together as in a bottle. They are separated and allotted different compartments throughout the body.

The closest fluid to the body's surface is the BLOOD. The water we drink is first taken up by the blood in the same way as oxygen is taken up by the lungs. However, blood constitutes only about 8% of the body's fluid. Surrounding the blood vessels and the body cells is a compartment that contains EXTRACELLULAR FLUID and lymph. These liquids constitute 22% of the body's fluids. They form the external environment of the body cells. They are like a pond in which the cells float. The extracellular fluids and lymph also circulate in the body. However, this circulation is much slower than blood circulation.

The deepest compartment of water in the body is the INTRACELLULAR FLUID or the water within the cells. It constitutes 70% of body's fluid. The cells acquire their solidity from the water that fills them in the same way as a tyre acquires its hardness from the air that fills it. When intracellular fluid becomes deficit, the cells lose their vitality and accumulate toxins.

The main function of water in the body is not merely to fill the empty spaces (its structural role), but also to carry nutrients like oxygen, glucose, minerals, etc. to the cells and remove their waste products (its transporter role). Water performs this transporter role through OSMOSIS.

3. What is Osmosis?

Osmosis occurs when two containers of liquid are separated by a permeable membrane or tissue. The dissolved solids exert an 'osmotic pressure' upon the membrane. It causes water to move from the least concentrated solution to the more concentrated solution until the pressure on both sides of the membrane is equalised. Some membranes are semi-permeable or have selective permeability. They allow certain substances like glucose, minerals, etc. to pass through. The movement of the dissolved substances is naturally in the direction opposite to the flow of water.

The cell membranes are semi-permeable and allow Potassium to enter, but they restrict the entry of Sodium and Chlorine. Hence, salt is largely found in the extracellular fluids and blood, and not within the cells. However, the cells can draw in Sodium from the intercellular fluid when it is necessary through the 'cellular pump' mechanism.

4. How does the water and nutrients pass through the body?

Water is largely absorbed in the upper portion of the small intestines through osmosis. The osmotic pressure of blood is normally higher, and hence water is easily transferred from the intestines through the capillaries into the blood stream. However, after meals the osmotic pressure of the blood is lower, and hence it is easier for the nutrients to pass into the blood.

The water that enters the blood dilutes it and reduces its osmotic pressure. In the other compartment of the body there are extracellular fluids, whose concentration of dissolved substances is quite close to that of the blood. This similarity enables the blood to transfer water, glucose, etc. to the extracellular fluids and also clear up the waste products from them.

The extracellular fluid ultimately transfers the nutrients to the cells. This also happens by osmosis or with the help of special tiny 'cell pumps' that are scattered over the surface of the cells. The cell pumps can monitor the flow of water, nutrients and waste products to and from the cells by a process similar to 'reverse osmosis'.

The body waste is ultimately collected by the blood and excreted along with water through the kidneys, lungs, glands in the skin, and the large intestines. The amount of water excreted through these channels can vary, but usually the volume that is passed as urine is 60%, as sweat is 20%, through the breath is 15%, and from the intestines is 5%.

5. What harm is caused by dehydration?

People can survive six weeks without food, but it is difficult to survive six days without water. Let us see what happens when the body is deprived of water:

First, the blood volume shrinks. Since it no longer receives water from the intestines, it draws water from the extracellular fluids. In the next stage the cells have insufficient fluid around them, and hence their functioning becomes intermittent and incomplete.

If the dehydration continues further, the extracellular liquid becomes thicker, and that makes the osmotic exchange with the blood and the cells more difficult. To remedy this situation, the cells are forced to give up some of their intracellular fluid. As a result the cells shrink and lose their vitality.

6. What happens when the body fluids become thicker?

Biological transformations in the body are performed by enzymes. However, the enzymes do not function properly when the body fluids have become more viscous. As a result the production of hormones, energy and reparative substances in the body is disturbed. Gradually, the urine becomes thicker, the sweat gets more concentrated and the stools become hard and dry. Ultimately, the rate of elimination of waste materials from the body is reduced and the condition of toxaemia arises – the body begins to suffocate from its own wastes.

7. What is the difference between acute and chronic dehydration?

Normally people think of dehydration as something that happens to people in the desert. However, something of a lesser intensity happens to people when their water intake is habitually less. In such a case most of the available water is taken by the vital organs and it becomes insufficient for other organs. Ultimately, the weakest link gives way, and that is where the disorder usually manifests itself.

8. What are some of the usual disorders associated with dehydration?

Fatigue

Once the enzyme activity in the body slows down, there is an underperformance of the enzymes associated with the production of energy. It gives rise to symptoms like lassitude, loss of energy and lack of enthusiasm.

Constipation

When too much liquid is withdrawn from the large intestines, constipation arises.

Digestive Disorders

Dehydration reduces the secretion of digestive juices. Hence, the digestion suffers. It gives rise to symptoms like bloating, nausea, acidity and loss of appetite.

Blood Pressure

In the normal course the blood is not sufficient at all places in the body. It is shifted around and made available where it is most needed. The body does this by selectively contracting the blood vessels.

Chronic dehydration reduces the volume of blood available and makes it thicker. Many blood vessels remain contracted so that there will be no shortage of blood where it is most needed. Over a period of time this 'defensive vasoconstriction' continues, and the arteries simply raise the blood pressure to push thicker blood through the blood vessels and compensate for the slowing down in the circulation. So, where the blood vessels are in a good tone and contract easily, there is hypertension or 'High BP'.

Where the vasoconstriction capacity is weak and the volume of blood shrinks, the blood vessels do not shrink enough to restrict the blood from flowing to places other than where it is most needed. That gives rise to the phenomena of slower circulation and 'Low BP'.

Respiratory disorders

When the respiratory mucus membranes dry out, they become less permeable to gaseous exchange. Then there is congestion and the lungs become susceptible to infections.

Skin Troubles

When chronic dehydration sets in the skin is unable to clear its toxins effectively. The skin cells become loaded with toxins and become prone to infections. Further, the thicker secretions cause foul odours and itching. There may be excessive scaling like dandruff or oozing like eczema.

High Cholesterol

Cholesterol performs various functions in the body and is involved in the construction of cell membranes. It serves the function of clay that makes the membranes semi-permeable or less permeable. Thus, there is a constant need for cholesterol in the blood.

Normally 1/3 of the cholesterol comes from food and 2/3 of it is produced in the liver and intestines. Hence, more often excess cholesterol is due to internal over production. Let us see how chronic dehydration increases the production of cholesterol in the body.

Once there is a chronic deficiency of water in the intracellular fluid, the body produces more cholesterol to make the cell membranes less permeable (so that they lose less water). However, this higher level of cholesterol has certain undesirable effects on the blood vessels. If you regulate the water level in the body, the body will generate signals that automatically reduce the cholesterol level in the blood, without requiring significant changes in your diet.

Rheumatism

When there is a higher level of toxins in the blood, some of them are absorbed by the joint cartilages and tissues. Then the joints become stiff and painful.

9. Is the need for water in the body regulated by the sensation of thirst?

The sensation of thirst normally indicates that you need to drink water. However, there are two kinds of needs, and they depend on whether the body is deficit in extracellular fluid and blood, or in intracellular fluid.

When there is a shortage of water in the blood or extracellular fluid, it may not be quenched by merely drinking water. Here, in addition to water, the body needs salt to retain the increase in water intake. This kind of thirst arises due to the summer heat or due to excessive athletic activity. There is excessive loss of water and salt (through perspiration). Such thirst can also arise due to persistent vomiting or diarrhoea. In such a case, you need to drink water with a little salt.

Intracellular deficiency of water can arise when the cells are made to part with their water to the extracellular fluid. This could arise due to a lack of water intake, but it could also be due to an excess of dissolved solids or salt in the blood, as after a meal. In both these cases, the thirst is quenched by drinking soft water without salt or minerals. Contrary to the belief that digestive juices are diluted by water consumed during meals, one glass should be consumed during meals to maintain the osmotic pressure that is necessary to move the food forward into the blood. You can allow the sensation of thirst to indicate the need.

Sometimes our sensation of thirst becomes confused due to habitual consumption of beverages, soft-drinks and alcoholic drinks. In such cases simply follow the water regime given below and the defect will autocorrect. In addition to the regime, we also make you aware of other properties of water so that you can consume the right kind of water.

10. How much water do we need to consume every day for rehydration?

The amount of water you need to consume will depend on your body weight and the seasons.

Under moderate climatic conditions a person doing office work would have the following needs: Weight 100 lbs or 45 kg needs 6 glasses (225 ml each) of water; 125 lbs or 56 kg needs 7 ½ glasses; 150 lbs or 67 kg needs 9 glasses; 175 lbs or 79 kg needs 10 ½ glasses; and 200 lbs or 90 kg needs 12 glasses. This is in addition to the two glasses you would consume with the meals.

The amount of water intake can be increased by 20% in summer and reduced by 20% in winter.

Water taken during meals, as beverages, soft-drinks, milk, etc. does not contribute significantly to detoxification. A simple water regime would be to take two glasses of water after waking, one glass of water a half-hour before every meal and two hours after every meal.

Here is a TIME TABLE for consuming nine glasses of water, which is in addition to the glass you normally consume during lunch and dinner:

6 am (2); 7.30 am (1); breakfast 8 am; 10 am (1);
12 noon (1);
lunch 1 pm, 3 pm (1); 5 pm (1); 6 pm (1); dinner 7 pm;
9 pm (1).

Further, since your daily intake of water by this regime is increased from the usual six glasses to nine glasses of water, you may need to consume more salt, particularly if you are using soft (RO) water or it is the hot season. You can do that by putting a pinch of salt and a few drops of lemon juice into the water you drink in the morning. Still further, if you are habituated to consuming beverages, consider taking them with the meals.

The effect of long standing dehydration cannot be overcome in a few days. This water regime must be continued for at least two months to see the results. During this treatment some symptoms of the older ailments may re-surface. Consider these symptoms to be a part of the healing process that is happening, and do not treat them with drugs. Just persist with the water regime and they will ultimately disappear on their own.

If you find it inconvenient to follow the timetable, prepare the amount of water you plan to drink in advance and take it with you. Then all you have to do is to finish it before the end of the schedule. Another way to remember to drink water is to replenish it every time you urinate.

11. What is provocative detoxification?

Here you generate some dehydration before rehydrating.

During the dry phase the blood loses water, but does not receive it from the food. Hence, it draws from the extracellular fluid, which in turn draws it from the intracellular fluid.

In the wet phase you not only compensate for loss of water in the cells, but also flush the cells with an excess. This is helpful in flushing the toxins out from the cells. You can do this practice for one day in a week. It is rejuvenating. However, you should not undertake this practice when your health is already weak.

The steps

The dry phase: Take a sauna bath or a long walk in the sun to induce heavy sweating. Immediately before or during this phase do not drink any water.

The wet phase: After inducing heavy sweating, drink one to two litres of water. Do it slowly, over a period of an hour. If the sweating was too profuse, add a pinch of salt to the water intake.

12. What is 'living water' and 'dead water'?

Water that flows in fast flowing rivers and streams is tossed around a lot. It charges the water with an abundant amount of 'life-force' or 'prana'. This prana is deficient in water that flows in cement canals and in pipes. Stagnant water from storage tanks has usually lost its prana.

A vortex of water is formed in fast flowing water, which collects a lot of prana. This type of water is known to give good results in agriculture. That is perhaps the reason why vegetation flourishes along the riverside. On the other hand, 'dead water' gives poor vegetation and it is not helpful in rejuvenating the bodily functions. When dead water is drunk the feeling of SLOSH arises in the stomach.

Further, water has memory. So the water that is purified through RO filtration may have removed all the dangerous chemicals, but the negative vibrations that were generated by these toxic substances remain in the water. Hence, once water is contaminated with pollutants it should be considered as dead for drinking purposes. Modern sewage treatment facilities can purify the water, but they cannot revive it.

13. How to recognise 'living water'?

Place a drop of mountain-spring water and tap water side by side and observe it under a microscope. The structure and shape will be completely different. The mountain-spring water will show a harmonious circular membrane around the drop. The drop formation will look like a pearl. The tap water will show a deformed membrane and a damaged outline.

Next, allow both the drops to DRY up and examine the pattern of the residue under a microscope or a magnifying glass. The mountain-spring water will show a grid structure or a pattern, whereas the tap water will show no pattern and will be like a heap of dust particles.

14. Are there any other properties of 'live water'?

Some scientists have observed the direction of spin of water molecules. Dead water is said to have a right or clockwise spin, whereas mountain-spring water is said to have a left or anticlockwise spin. The healing water of 'Lourdes' in France and the 'Ganges water' in India are said to have a left spin.

Based on this observation people have devised 'REVITALIZER MACHINES' that are capable of inducing a left spin. They energise the water by generating a vortex motion. The anti-clockwise spin is generated by passing the water from one bottle to another through a small hole. Flush the toilet and see the flow. It is the same principle. They turn the bottle upside down and shake it. The water forms an anticlockwise vortex as it flows from one bottle to another.

Perhaps a more convenient way to energise water is to pass it through air by pouring it from one glass to another to 'PRANA-ATE' it. The energised water will be more refreshing than ordinary tap water. Another way to generate the left spin is to put filtered water into a kitchen blender and spin it for a few seconds. It will give it an anti-clockwise spin for a few seconds. This water can be stored in a non-metallic container and consumed during the day. However, it is best to consume bottled mountain-stream water

B. Baths & Packs

People are aware of the function of the skin in conveying sensations and regulating the body temperature. However, many people are not sufficiently aware of the other functions of the skin – *it breathes, absorbs some applications and excretes waste.* Skin is the biggest organ of the body and an excellent eliminator of toxins from the body. Let us see how this fact is utilised in nature cure.

1. Cleansing baths

In a cleansing bath water is used not just to clean dirt from the body, but also to draw out toxins from it.

The bath basics:

The proper time for bathing is *before* breakfast. Avoid eating just before or after a bath.

First clean the body with warm water and soap. Then give it a *scrub or rub* the skin with your hands. It stimulates the activity of the skin.

End the shower with room temperature water. The skin pores must be shut with cool water *before* you come out of a bath.

While wiping your body, *pat it* dry with a towel and do not rub it dry. Further, don't dry the body completely. Use the *'non-drying method'* used by the yogis. Simply wear the under-clothes when the body is still moist. Then wear the outer clothes and walk around a bit to allow the body to dry from body motion. This practice invigorates the skin and stimulates its elimination capacity.

If you have good endurance, try bathing with room temperature water. The body's reaction to cold water strengthens the vitality. Regular practice of cold water bathing will make your skin rugged and strengthen your immune system. The trick in being able to take cold water bath lies in *warming* the body with exercise just *before* taking the bath.

2. Hasty hand baths

Normally the rule for visiting a meditation room or a temple is to bathe before entering. However, this is not always convenient. So, there is a short cut. Dip your hands into room-temperature water and then rub them hastily over your entire body. Then pat your body dry with your handkerchief.

This practice is not done for cleaning the dirt. It has an invigorating and toning effect on the entire body.

3. Floating organ bath

This practice is used to relax and rejuvenate the functions of the floating organs, namely the liver, kidneys, pancreas, and spleen.

Dip your body in a half full tub of water so that the abdomen is kept below the water level. You can pass the hand gently over the belly from time to time during the bath. It is very satisfying. The duration is 15 minutes.

4. Foot bath

This is used to overcome fatigue and the tired feeling before going to sleep. It calms the nerves and gives restful sleep.

Dip the feet into a half-filled bucket of mildly hot water. You can add some bath salts to spice things up. Keep the feet in water for ten minutes. Then take out the feet and pour room-temperature water over them and rub them as though you are washing off the toxins. Then pat them dry and keep them wrapped up in a blanket for about ten minutes.

5. Wet pack

Take a thin sheet of course linen or a sari and dip it in water. Next, squeeze the water out leaving the sheet moist. Then spread the sheet on the floor. Lie naked on the sheet and carefully wrap it around the body from neck to foot, like an Egyptian Mummy. First practice this. Then immediately have someone wrap a blanket around you and place a pillow under your head. Have them put another blanket over you.

Stay in the pack for 30 to 45 minutes. During this time you will sweat. Think that the body is eliminating the toxins. Then unwrap yourself and immediately take a cleansing bath. You must drink a large glass of water before packing yourself and after the bath. This method is very effective in drawing out the toxins from the cells deep below the skin.

6. Half pack

This method is similar to the wet pack, but here only half of the body, from the neck to the trunk, is wrapped.

This method is popular because it is very convenient. People who have a weak vital force should use it to strengthen themselves. This method is superior to sauna baths. If you use it regularly, once in a week, within one or two months your skin will become softer and velvety and it will begin to glow.

E. The Cleansing Diet

This diet has two considerations. The first consideration is to give our body a long period of rest from digestion on a daily basis. During the rest the body will use the extra energy to eliminate the toxins. The second consideration is to eat fruits with good cleansing properties in the morning (elimination time). It will assist the elimination effort.

The best cleansing fruits are Black Grapes, Pomegranate, Guava and Papaya. Other good fruits are Apples, Figs, Prunes, Jambu, Orange, Mango, Peach, Pears, Grapefruit, Chiku, and Dates. Citric fruits have cleansing properties, but people who suffer from rheumatic troubles should avoid consuming them. Banana can be difficult to digest. So, avoid eating banana during breakfast or dinner. Melons don't go well with other food. Hence, eat them alone.

Further, when you are on an elimination diet, don't do heavy body building exercises. You can take long walks and do yogic or aerobic exercises. This diet should show good results within two months.

F. The Therapeutic Fast

What cleansing diets can do in two months, fasting can do in just three days! Hence, if you are obese or if you have some long-standing disease, consider taking up a therapeutic fast for three days.

Before undertaking the fast, you should get ACCLIMATISED to the idea of the fast. *How can you do that?* Try to abstain from food for progressively longer hours. For example, begin by increasing the interval between meals. Avoid snacking between meals. Then go further: Miss one dinner or meal every week. This preparation is necessary before you undertake a therapeutic fast.

BEGIN the fast by taking only fruit for breakfast. Thereafter do not take any food on the second and third day. During the fast consume warm water, avoid excessive physical activity.

On the FOURTH DAY, break the fast by taking some fruits for breakfast. Don't overdo this. Take a snack meal for lunch. Then if you need more cleansing, continue with the cleansing diet. You can safely repeat the fast after a month.

Note that fasting is not starving! People can safely live for a few weeks without food. Hence, a fast of three is certainly not going to kill you. Instead, you will be amazed to see the body clean up the toxins and drugs that have been thrust upon it for years.

Some additional considerations:

a) Many SYMPTOMS can arise during a fast. For example: On the FIRST DAY, you will get restless at meal times. It is due to the habit of the body. If you are habituated to drinking beverages like tea or coffee, you may experience some 'withdrawal symptoms' like headache. The mind may also become restless and make you think only of food. Hence, you may find it difficult to focus on anything else. At such times, it is good to distract yourself. Watch TV, play some computer game, read a book or chat with friends.

b) On the SECOND and THIRD DAY, the hunger sensation will begin to dry up and the expectoration and bodily secretion will increase. They may become foul smelling. If you experience too much foul odour, you can take more baths with warm water. However, don't try to relieve these symptoms with tonics, glucose, vitamins or drugs. The foul discharges are actually a good sign, since they indicate that the healing process has begun. As the toxaemia reduces, the body odour will change, the tongue will become clearer, the skin will look healthier, your face and eyes will brighten up, your appetite will return, and you will feel healthier.

c) There may be a short 'healing or elimination crisis': You may experience some giddiness, purging, vomiting, fever, headache, rashes and foul odour. There may also be a regression, the reappearance of some symptoms of an old disease process. Some symptoms of an old illness may reappear and then slowly begin to fade away. *This elimination crisis is a part of the natural cleansing process, and it is usually followed by a strengthening of the vital force.* Thus, some of your symptoms of the ailment may get aggravated, but your overall health condition will continue to improve. At such times it is good to have a friend or partner around who is supportive of your fasting and cleansing.

d) On the FOURTH DAY break the fast by taking some fruit or fruit juice for breakfast. Then gradually increase the food intake with each meal.

G. 'Mono Fruit Diets' and 'Raw Vegetable Juice Diets'

Fasting is the chief remedy in naturopathy. Hence, many variations have been developed. They are interesting and cater to different needs. Further since you consume some fruit during the fast, the fast is not so severe.

Mono Fruit Diet

Here the fruits used are citrus fruit, black grapes or apple. Citrus fruits are used when the patient is susceptible to colds or has a mucus condition. However, it should be avoided if there is a tendency to rheumatic troubles or ulcers.

Black grapes are used for purifying the blood, when there is a heart condition or when the vitality is low.

Apples are used where there is rheumatic or inflammatory condition.

During these fruit diets you can eat the chosen fruit for all the meals, but do not take any other food. You can vary the amount of fruit intake according to your need, but do not overeat. The fast is usually taken for three to seven days.

Raw Vegetable Juice Diet

Here the vegetables used are carrots, cabbage or bottle gourd (dudhi). Such diets are used to correct digestive disorders and conditions like colitis and ulcers. Beet juice is used when the vitality is low.

H. The No-Breakfast Plans

Now we consider a variation of the elimination diet. It is based on the fact that when the vital force has become weak, it cannot effectively carry out the functions of digestion and elimination simultaneously. So when it is attending to digestion, the elimination is weak. The saying is: "Eat less to detoxify more". The aim of the no-breakfast plan is to give the body a long period *of rest from digestion on a daily basis*. When the no-breakfast becomes a habit, the body will use the extra vitality available at that time to eliminate the toxins. There are three variations of this plan.

Plan A: Don't eat anything for breakfast. Just drink a lot of water or take it with green tea or with a little lemon juice and salt.

Plan B: Eat only cleansing fruits for breakfast. These fruits require very little digestion and yet they give you the feeling of having eaten. So this kind of fast is easier to keep.

Plan C: Take oat-porridge with dry fruits like dates, figs and resins for breakfast. This plan is for those who find it difficult to follow Plan-B. The aim here is to eat the food that requires a minimum of digestion so that there is no load on digestion in the morning. Eat only little, so that you do not depress the sensation of hunger that should arise at lunch time.

The no-breakfast plan is the most practical fasting plan and it has given very consistent results. Just try it for a few months and you will see the marvellous results for yourself.

I. Schedule for Implementation

You do not get healthy by reading a book on health. You have to practice the methods and recommendations to reduce the toxaemia. Once the toxaemia comes under control, your health and immunity will most certainly improve.

So, let us implement the recommendations and methods you have learnt. The easiest way is to make a schedule and try to follow it. Here we suggest a schedule according to the seasons. We have used six seasons (Ayurvedic) instead of the usual four.

	Season	Months	Recommendation
1	Winter	Jan-Feb	No fasting
2	Spring	Mar-Apr	Elimination diet
3	Summer	May-Jun	Water therapy
4	Rainy	Jul-Aug	Fasting or Elimination diet
5	Interim (Sharad)	Sep-Oct	Elimination diet or Water therapy
6	Autumn	Nov-Dec	No fasting

Chapter-4:

The Hidden Causes of Disease

Yoga Vaisistha (my rendering): *Ignorance gives rise to absence of self-control. A person without self-control is constantly distracted by likes and dislikes, and by egoistic thoughts and personal considerations. Such a person becomes prone to all kinds of disturbances.*

The absence of mental restraint and improper living habits give rise to ailments in the body. Other causes are untimely and irregular activities, unhealthy habits, evil company and wicked thoughts. All these things weaken the energy channels (nadis) in the body and prevent the free flow of the life-force through them.

Health is a holistic concept. Healing does not merely consist of following some dietary habits. You have to *support* the diet with good living habits. And to do that you have to become more conscious of how you live. The body will provide the *feedback* on your mistakes. However, it is always up to you to recognise your mistakes and make the necessary adjustments in your thoughts and actions.

Once you accept the responsibility for your health, your task is to do what you can do to improve your health and simply accept what you cannot do. Genetic and toxic environmental factors are outside your control. Hence, you must accept these. However, your thoughts, emotions (reactions) and habits are under your will and you can exercise your control here. However, before you can exercise this control effectively you have to understand how you consciously or unconsciously participate in generating your ailments. To help you we consider below five causes or factors behind our illnesses.

- The Stress Factor

- The Psychosomatic Causes

- On handling emotions

- Healing by Changing the Consciousness

- The Karmic Causes

A. The Stress Factor

Stress is a term used by Holistic physicians to describe the human response to the difficulties of life. In modern times the stress factor has become a major contributor to diseases such as heart attacks, high BP, ulcers and nervous disorders. Compared to physical tensions, the emotional tensions are even more disruptive factors to health. Hence, it is important to study all this in detail.

1. What happens to the body under stress?

We normally think of ourselves as something that is living under the skin. What is outside the skin is something else, and it is a potential threat to what is inside. And, what is inside is ME! This sense of separation creates a *perpetual fear* in us. The fear makes us defensive and generates tension in our body.

Whenever we perceive a threat, our body gets into a stress response, and we experience the *'fight or flight syndrome'*: Our body gets ready for action. The *nervous system* becomes excited, the *muscles* contract, the *heart* pumps faster, and the *digestion* stops to provide excess circulation of blood to the muscular system and the *excretory system* discharges (urine, stools, sweat, etc.)

Thus, tension is a *defence mechanism* of the body. It makes us ready for quick short-term action. This reaction is a fitting response to a challenge in the JUNGLE where we have to fight or run away. However, in modern society we are faced with different kinds of SITUATIONS LIKE a traffic jam, a lawyer's notice, having to speak before an audience, work deadlines, bad boss, cash flow problems, social and marriage problems, emotional problems, self-esteem issues, etc. The stress response, which is helpful in the jungle, does not help in such situations. There is worry (fear of uncertainty) and anxiety (fear of the unknown), and these factors put us under continuous pressure. The 'stress response' in these conditions is wasteful. What is needed is a more thoughtful approach that can prepare us for long term action.

Our modern lifestyle adds much to our tensions. It keeps us perpetually dissatisfied. We become greedy and try to do too much or want results very quickly. Hence, there is a lot of rushing about for nothing.

If the stress response is allowed to continue in the body, it gives rise to CHRONIC TENSION — we stay in the over-prepared condition for a long period of time. Then our energy reserves get depleted and we get into an EXHAUSTED STATE. On the *psychological level*, our awareness becomes constricted (we become impatient and don't see other people's concerns too well), and this often makes us aggressive, irritable or quarrelsome. On the *physical level*, we develop many stress-related disorders (reactions) such as allergies, high BP, heart disease, headaches, ulcers, chronic indigestion, dandruff, eczema and insomnia.

Let us begin by recognizing the *signs* of our physical and emotional tensions. Then we shall observe the typical *symptoms* of tension in the body. And ultimately we shall learn how to *deal* with the causes.

2. What are the physical signs of tension?

When you get into the stress response the MUSCLES get tense, the jaw tightens and the heart beats rapidly. The NERVES become excited and you become shaky or fidgety. The BLOOD is withdrawn from the digestion process, and hence the mouth becomes dry. The blood flows away from the skin, and hence you develop dry skin and dandruff. The excitement may cause the SKIN to throw out the moisture, and that gives rise to excessive or profuse perspiration. The body wants to REDUCE its load, and hence the stools and the urine are discharged. Prolonged tension can exhaust the EYE muscles. Then, the pupils remain dilated and it causes night blindness.

3. What are the emotional signs of tension?

The stress response makes you defensive. So, you hold on to things or react vehemently as though you have been threatened. (This can cause constipation or diarrhoea). It can make you UPTIGHT so you FEAR the people or situations that do not normally bother others, or you can become unnecessarily SUSPICIOUS of others.

The emotional tension makes it difficult for you to take joy from the small pleasures of everyday living. Even small problems and disappointments can throw you into utter confusion. Or you become emotionally FRAGILE and are quick to take offence. Usually, you find it HARD TO 'LET GO' of any wrong that was done to you. If the emotional tension is allowed to continue for long, you can sink into DEPRESSION. Then, you feel inadequate and doubt your ability to cope with your situation.

We live in a society where we constantly experience many POWER STRUGGLES: It may be a struggle in our male-female relationships, in the office with a colleague or even with a friend or acquaintance. This struggle expresses itself in many ways: We try to get our way; we always want to be right; we don't value another person's opinion; or we feel the need to criticise others or put them down. All such signs show that we lack personal power.

The causes of emotional stress hide in your SUBCONSCIOUS. Hence, to know them you have to dig them out. You may find the cause to be due to some emotional injury, an unfulfilled emotional need, a disappointment in a relationship, some let-down, an unfulfilled ambition or simply a disappointment with yourself. Further, the cause may be due to a setback or trauma in your childhood, a feeling of rejection, some disempowering belief, a feeling of being violated, a feeling of worthlessness, or simply the fear of failure.

4. What are the typical symptoms of stress?

When the tension is allowed to continue for a long time, the mental and bodily FUNCTIONS get disturbed. *Then what happens?* Either you EAT too much (nervously) or you experience a loss of appetite (due to poor circulation). The NERVES remain in an excited condition and therefore you develop insomnia or disturbed sleep. And if that is allowed to continue, you get into an *'exhausted state'*.

Then you become reactive, irritable, and forgetful. It may make you hypersensitive, quarrelsome and intolerant of other people's habits; or you may become restless, indecisive, and have difficulty in concentrating on anything.

Many people try to come out of this state of continuous tension, by slipping into external *dependencies* like smoking, drinking, sex and consuming beverages.

5. How can you overcome stress in daily life?

Whenever you see yourself get into the stress response (when the heart begins to throb rapidly, the muscles contract and you become impatient or hyper tense), introduce a deliberate calm in your body.

You can do this by doing some deep belly-breathing, by meditating, or by chanting a mantra until the stress eases. The method is not as important as using it as often as necessary.

6. Some strategies to reduce physical stress

To overcome physical stress you have to make adjustments in your LIFE-STYLE: You have to overcome the subconscious *habit of staying busy* and constantly doing something or living under the *constant pressure* of having to succeed or perform. In particular:

- Make realistic plans. Don't try to DO MORE than you can. Allow some transition time between the activities.
- Don't wait for things to become urgent or overdue. Allot time to things that are IMPORTANT to you. Start them a little earlier than you have to.
- Your time and energy are always limited. Hence, you cannot keep on adding activities to your life. You have to make some SUBSTITUTIONS. So, from time to time, review your routine activities, and eliminate the inessential and the unwanted. Otherwise, you'll precipitate a crisis.
- SLOW DOWN the pace of your life so that you can act MORE INTENTIONALLY — with greater awareness and care.

7. How to handle emotional stress?

First become fully aware of the emotional factors you need to deal with. In many cases you may have to dig this out to make an accurate diagnosis.

After you know the emotional factors and the harmful effect they are having on you, make a conscious decision to close the 'open wounds' of your life. Simply bring the emotional factor forward in your mind. Do it one at a time. Then expel it with your will. 'Let go' of it once and for all.

How do you know that you have let go of it? When you have done that you will not feel the subconscious urge to react or back-bite any more.

8. Some common lifestyle habits that reduce stress

Sleep Well:

Do not compromise on your sleep. You need seven to eight hours of sound sleep daily to replenish your vitality. Further, the replenishing value of sleep is not the same at all times. Two hours of sleep before midnight is equivalent to four hours of sleep after midnight. Hence, go to sleep early and wake up early.

Take Exercise:

Take a long walk every morning to improve your circulation and promote the elimination of toxins. Walk in a rhythm. Choose a quiet and open space for the walk. In between the walk take a break and sit quietly under a tree or on a bench for a few minutes. Try to enjoy the peace.

Don't Be Rushed:

Do not rush through your life or try to do too much. Learn to say 'no' to things that you don't have time for or that don't deserve your attention. Do just a few things, but take the satisfaction of doing them well.

Avoid Reacting:

You subconsciously interpret the information you come across based on the desires, fears and tendencies in your mind. These interpretations cause you to take things personally and to react to what has happened. When the reactions are strong, you disturb the energies (emotions) in the body and generate toxins.

You can overcome this habit of the mind by learning to look upon the happenings of life disinterestedly. If there is something you can do in a situation, proceed to do it. However, when you cannot do anything about the situation, let it pass and simply refuse to react to it. When you do that, you don't 'bottle up' the life-force with emotional knots.

Don't carry grudges or injured feelings:

Become aware of the emotional wounds from your past that you are still carrying. Then resolve to deliberately close them. Consider that what happened was relevant only within that context. Now the context has changed, and hence the old emotions are 'out of place'. They must be rejected.

Live Spiritually:

Live to serve a purpose that is larger than your self-interest. Always try to include others in your personal agenda. Let your personal benefit arise out of the benefit that you bring to others.

If you keep up this practice, it will change the focus of your life. Then, instead of being 'ego centred' you will become 'principle centred'. It will relieve you of the 'burden' of your personal life.

B. The Psychosomatic Causes

Normally, when we think in terms of cure, we assume that something external can be taken to treat something that is happening within the body. This assumption is okay when we are treating infections, but when the cause of the ailment is within our system, as in our mind, to treat it with external agents like drugs or surgery is very indirect. You can only relieve some effects or symptoms in this way. To heal the person we have to deal with the causes inside the person. When that is done, the 'diseased state' gets transformed. Then the recovery can be remarkable.

1. Aren't psychosomatic disorders treated by drugs?

Psychiatrists use drugs to treat depression, anxiety and distress. But these drugs do not cure or transform the person. They simply disconnect (sedate) the person temporarily from the inner turmoil. Drugs or surgical measures relieve or sedate some symptoms of the malady, but they cannot heal or restore normalcy in the person. And when people take such treatment, the will power, which needs to be strengthened, is weakened further. Hence, the psychiatric approach to treating psychosomatic disorders is inappropriate. The correct approach is to find or recognise the inner cause and relieve it.

2. What is the role of trauma in such diseases?

To know the psychosomatic cause behind an ailment you have to look deeper into the emotional side of life. In many cases the cause is due to a TRAUMA – a major damaging psychological event that had occurred in the life of a person. The effect of a trauma is not merely psychological. It generates emotions that continue to brew in the subconscious. And from there these emotions maintain psychological complexes and 'energy locks' within the body. Unless you release these energy locks and expel the emotions that are causing them, the emotions will continue to generate ailments in the mind and the nervous system. The traumas experienced during the younger years of life often develop into serious ailments in the later years. However, people ignore this cause because it is difficult to see the connections between the root cause and the ultimate effects.

In Pranic healing the effect of a trauma is often sensed as an energy depression in the chest. This energy has to be cleansed and recharged. When that is done, the trauma impression re-surfaces and the patient becomes aware of the cause. Then the patient can be encouraged to release the impressions they have been carrying so that no more harmful emotions are generated.

3. The psychosomatic causes of certain disorders

The following discussion on the causes of psychosomatic ailments is only suggestive. You can use it to understand the nature of the causes that underlie such ailments. However, it should not be used to brand or categorise any patient. Further, don't push these generalisations on people who are in a 'denial mode'. They are simply not yet ready to face up to such knowledge. If you press them into making admissions, you only increase their pain instead of relieving it.

To make good use of this chapter, you must not consider your ailment as a 'chance happening'. There is a cause, and it is in your nature; and if you look for it you will find it. You must know the cause before you look for ways to overcome it. Further, in finding the ways you should be tentative and experimental. If something is not working, try something else that works. Very often you will need to make some changes in your attitude and lifestyle. In any case, once you have understood the cause you have to act. The psychosomatic disorders always thrive on your inaction and excuses!

Accidents

Our preoccupation with fear, greed or anger leads to inattention or carelessness; which precipitates accidents.

Addictions

When the will power is weak or when the person's self-esteem or self-worth is seriously damaged, it causes the person to take the support of some external dependency, like smoking or drinking.

Negative thoughts and behavioural patterns are also forms of addiction. For example, we can become addicted to losing our temper or to begging for sympathy.

Alzheimer's disease

This arises due to degeneration in the part of the brain associated with memory. However, more often it happens because the mind begins to die earlier than the body. The increasing prevalence of this disease in modern times is understandable since the elders, who were once respected and considered to be the custodians of wisdom, are now treated as dependents or unwanted family members. They experience chronic insecurity, fear of rejection, fear of being abandoned and fear of becoming institutionalised.

Technology has lengthened life, but it has not helped in improving the value of the person!

Allergies or diseases of the Immune System

The immune system is sensitive to both viruses from outside and emotions from the inside. It is strengthened when you 'feel safe' emotionally. On the other hand, when we have unstable relationships, single parent households, broken homes, or we feel victimised the instability factor increases.

The chief aggravating factor in allergies is irritation – with oneself, with other people or with life. The typical disorders are common cold, influenza, herpes, etc.

Arthritis

It is associated with rigid thinking and beliefs or sometimes simply being afraid of being flexible.

Back Pains

The back is the main support system of the body. When we fear the lack of support, feel unsupported by others, or feel incapable of supporting ourselves, the back gives in. Problems in the upper back show a lack of love or emotional support, whereas problems in the lower back are related to a lack of physical or material support.

Colon Disorders

Here the lack of self-confidence is internalised to give frequent motions, whereas irritation about someone or something gives constipation.

Diabetes

One form of it arises from the internalization of the responsibility issue – the resentment of having to take care of another person. Sometimes it is due to a lack of sweetness (joy) in our life.

(Chronic) Fatigue

This is certainly aggravated by a feeling of hopelessness or helplessness. Sometimes it is due to a trauma, some setback or loss.

Female Sexual Problems

This is often due to anger or resentment against having a female body, about being a woman, or being against living in a male dominated society.

(Weak) Hands

Our hands represent our ability to reach out or to grasp things. Hands become weak when we lack this ability. When we are unwilling or afraid to receive, it can make the left hand susceptible. And when we cannot give, it can make the right hand susceptible.

Heart Troubles

The heart is very sensitive to a lack of affection. When the heart is affected we are afraid or unwilling to trust or love openly.

Kidney Trouble

Kidney problems are due to internalization of irritation and fear.

(Weak) Legs

Being self-reliant, standing firm and being grounded are related. When there is fear in this connection, the feet are affected.

Liver Trouble

Internalization of anger affects the liver. Sometimes it is due to the suppressed feeling of injustice. Such feelings generate biliousness or hot toxins.

Neck Problem

The neck is always affected by stress. A stiff neck is associated with rigidity or with clinging on to our thoughts or ideas.

Pain

Pain is often caused by suppressed fear (anxiety or worry). It is easier to say: "*My back hurts*" than to say: "*My marriage or job hurts.*" Often, people continue to 'feel' the hurt to attract sympathy.

Sometimes the internalisation of frustration also causes pain.

Panic Attacks

These happen because we sense inadequacy, fear competition, fear of being replaced, etc.

4. How psychosomatic disorders are regarded

The medical profession has more or less ignored the psychosomatic cause and the public tends to interpret it as a 'personality flaw'. Hence, the society usually ignores this factor until it becomes really unmanageable or untreatable.

Who si prone to psychosomatic disorders? The individual who harbours a lot of dissatisfaction and discontentment in their life are more prone to having such disorders.

5. Do you have to make some inner changes to overcome your psychosomatic ailment?

When you have a common cold, you can tell yourself: *"A cold is not a cold to me but it is nature's way to tell – that I have been eating lately not wisely but too well!"* In the same way, when you have emotional troubles, do not seek external solutions. Don't say, *"You don't love me (trust me, visit me, etc.) as much as before."* Ask yourself, *"Why should they?"* Are you really as lovable, as trustworthy, or as interesting as before? Find the flaw in your thinking and correct it. If you don't do it, the problem won't solve itself.

Many people think that looking to the inner life and finding the emotional causes of your troubles there is very difficult work. Further, to get results you have to change how you regard some things or respond to them. However, this 'inner work' is only as difficult as you make it. You can always use the help of a guide. He or she can help you in making the change a gradual process – by showing you how you can climb in small steps over a period of time.

6. Can the mind-body relationship be used for self-healing?

Just as disease can be the result of negative thinking and emotions, positive thinking can be used to restore health. When your mind gets into a negative mode, your vital force gets disturbed. And that makes you prone to diseased states. In the same way, when your mind gets into a positive mode the vital forces gets energised. Then you develop immunity from diseased states.

Hence, you should keep the company of happy people, and good thoughts (like thoughts of hope, courage and confidence). Happiness is contagious and it promotes health.

C. On handling emotions

1. The nature of emotions

Emotions are like shadows — they have an amplifying effect. When they arise in the mind they make your problem appear to be much more or much less than it is. So, when you are driven by emotions, you easily get upset by difficulties or elated by hope or opportunities. The emotions create an unbalanced condition in your mind that makes you either pessimistic or optimistic.

The common emotions you have to deal with will be related to your self-esteem and other personal considerations.

2. Your interpretations make you emotional

Something happens, and then subconsciously you interpret this information according to the desires, fears and tendencies in your mind. These interpretations cause you to take things very personally.

If the reactions are strong, your vital force gets disturbed and begins to malfunctions. Then functional disorders arise in your body.

However, you can overcome the subconscious habit to over-react.. You can do it by adopting a non-reactive point of view to the happenings of life. If there is something you can do in a situation, you can try to do it. Otherwise you t let the situation pass WITHOUT generating personal reactions to it. When you can practice this, you don't 'bottle up' your life-force with emotional knots.

3. How to avoid generating personal reactions?

You do it by creating a GAP between a thought that arises in the mind and your emotional interpretation of it. The interpretation is a second or subsequent thought. When you understand this, you can separate the thoughts and put a wedge between them. Now you can re-examine the first thought objectively and look upon it impersonally.

You can go further and try to balance the after-thoughts that have arisen in your mind. It this way you overcome the habit of taking a one-sided view of things. When your interpretations are balanced, your emotions subside naturally. Then they cannot disturb your perceptions. Then you can observe everything objectively and know what is true.

D. Healing by Changing your Consciousness

1. How we become susceptible to disease

The prototype or original model of the human body in consciousness is perfect and healthy. Then, why does susceptibility to disease and constitutional disorders arise in our body?

They arise largely from certain defective patterns that we carry in our mindset. We have inherited some of these patterns from our previous existence, and some of them are the result of our actions in the present existence. Our consciousness gets associated with the contents of our mind, which are the personal thoughts, disturbing emotions, compulsive tendencies and faulty beliefs. And this association creates faults in the consciousness of our vital force or prana of the body. This faulty or disturbed prana then becomes ineffective in maintaining our body in a healthy condition, and gradually functional and constitutional disorders begin to arise in it.

Thus, the contents of our mind are largely responsible for the diseases in our body. The good news is that the effects are reversible. By making some changes in our belief-system, tendencies and negative emotions we carry in our subconscious, we can restore the consciousness of our vital force. Then it will restore health in our mind and body.

2. The way

Since our vital force is the true healer, the healing power is within us; and in its natural condition it is sufficient to maintain our health. The vital force malfunctions due to the negative patterns and entities in our mind. We are not sufficiently conscious of these patterns and entities, and so we allow them to disturb our vital force, influence our actions, and maintain our bad habits.

The negative patterns and emotions arise when we consider the happenings in life from a very personal and egoistic point of view. If we replace our point of view with a spiritual consciousness – with a large hearted and inclusive point of view, the consciousness in the vital force will get restored, and it will be able to perform its natural function of healing our body.

3. Live the truth of health

Your health is holistic, so you are never sick in a part. The part is only the place where the ailment has shown up. It is always a mistake to focus on repairing a part of the body in isolation of the mental mechanism (thoughts and emotions) that has caused the ailment.

So, the major task in healing through consciousness is to FIND the deep-seated patterns caused by your egoistic considerations and to REPLACE them with the patterns got from a spiritual consciousness. The new patterns will make you large hearted and bring kindness, courage and joy into your life; it will change the consciousness in the vital force and cells of the body. And health will be the natural outcome.

Once you have lost your health, the restoration doesn't happen automatically. You have to develop a health consciousness and allow it change your habits and lifestyle, and clear the negative emotions from your subconscious. In short, you have to promote your 'health consciousness'; and let your actions speak louder than your words. Then your health consciousness will make you healthy.

4. A Practice: Choose what you think

Pause often during the day to *hear the self-talk* going on inside your mind. These are the personal thoughts and psychological memories repeating themselves. They arise due to your egoistic point of view.

Now change your point of view: Decide to live and work for a cause that is always greater than your selfishness and personal considerations. Then your task is to look upon everything from higher point of view, and to reject the thoughts and self-talk that arises from a selfish and personal point of view. That's all.

Choose the thoughts you want to think, and reject the negative thoughts that want to do your thinking. Accept one and reject the other; and do it persistently. Gradually this practice will change your consciousness.

5. Affirmations for good health

Your health mirrors your convictions. Hence, if you are constantly ill, you do not believe wholeheartedly in perfect health. So, take this opportunity to install some healthy beliefs in your mind. Declare these statements to yourself:

a) "Wellness is my natural state."

b) "I am now filled with the energy of life."

c) "My body will serve me as long as I need it. Hence, I banish the idea of old-age problems or going to an infirmary."

d) "I am now healthy, energetic, enthusiastic and peaceful."

Next, try to ACT AS THOUGH your health is real. Do it even if you are not really healthy.

6. Some necessary points of view

a) *The original nature of the human body does not have sickness*. Hence, my sickness is due to personal factors that disturb the natural flow of life-energy (*prana*) in my body.

b) *My world is the result of my consciousness projected on a screen.* Hence, I do not have to do workouts to develop a healthy body. I have to only develop a health consciousness to become healthy.

c) If I fear disease or poverty, I have a disease or poverty consciousness. It is sufficient to make me sick or poor. However, *if I have faith in God and try to serve the spiritual purpose of my life, I develop a peaceful and loving consciousness*. It is sufficient to make me happy.

6. Changing the consciousness in organs

Although there is a whole body consciousness, there is also a 'whole organ consciousness' — that is each organ also has its own consciousness. You can speak to an organ and change its consciousness. Many disorders in the organs can be corrected in this way.

Consider the situation to be like this: Some cells of an organ have become lazy or rebellious. They are like 'rebellious mind-bits' that are cross or 'out-of-sorts'. Then you can directly connect with their consciousness and call upon them to change. You can scold them or coax them into performing the right action. Just speak mentally to the 'cell-minds' in the same way as you would talk to under-developed children. Tell to them what you expect them to do. Here are some examples:

To treat frequent STOMACH disorders:

Tap the stomach and say as follows: "*Wake up. You are neglecting your work. You have to ensure that everything I put in is digested properly. Now show me that you can do it.*" Give this order daily for a few days to see the results.

To treat LIVER troubles:

Speak to the organ as above. However, the liver is the domain of Saturn. Hence, its mind is dull and stupid. You have to speak to it firmly and positively. You cannot coax it into action; you must demand it. You can also talk to the liver in the case of frequent constipation (deficiency of bile) and diarrhoea (excess of bile).

To treat frequent RHEUMATIC disorders:

Excessive toxins like uric acid in the blood make the joints and ligaments prone to rheumatic disorders. Then you have to reduce the toxaemia in the body. But to help in relieving the trouble, speak to the stiff joint. Ask it to relax and push out the toxins that are making it stiff. However, in addition to the specific joint, you should treat the kidneys. The minds of kidney cells are similar to the liver, but they are more rebellious. Sometimes, you may need to talk to the stomach and ask it to produce less acid.

To treat HEART trouble:

The heart is a very sensitive organ. Hence, it responds to loving instructions. Speak to its consciousness with loving care, and it will respond.

To treat ANY bodily trouble

Give a positive suggestion of health and relaxation to the vital force and displaces the thought of illness. It will facilitate the healing.

E. The Karmic Causes

The karmic causes of an ailment arise from the mistakes in our actions (thinking included). These are of two kinds – acts against our conscience and acts against others or the principle of unity. Such actions generate conflicts within us, and these internal conflicts further become the cause of our misfortune and ailments.

1. What is the consequence of a conflict against our conscience?

When we act against our conscience, we get divided internally. Then we are unable to control our desires or urges, and we are unable to do what we believe to be correct.

The saying is: "*Our body and mind belong to the Soul, our inner being, in the same way as our horse or house belongs to us.*" Hence, when we live for the sake of pleasurable sensations or the ambitions of our ego, we cannot act according to our perception of truth. Instead, if we follow the voice of our conscience, we experience a truth-sense, which will guide us in all the situations of our life.

2. What is the consequence of conflicting with others?

A conflict between our mind and other minds results in disharmony. All of us are connected on the inner planes, and the influences go both ways. Disharmony creates imbalance and tensions in our mind, and that makes us 'out of sorts'. On the other hand, if we uphold the thought of togetherness, kindness, interdependence and peace, it becomes easier for us to find the right things to do in society. When our actions are based on this harmony, we generate health and prosperity.

Dr. Edward Bach (well known for 'floral remedies') suggests that there is a relationship between a disharmony and a bodily ailment. For example: **Pride** gives rise to rigidity and stiffness in the body; **cruelty** to others gives rise to pain; **hatred** gives rise to loneliness, short-temper and hysteria; **self-love** or over concern about oneself gives rise to neurosis (obsession and depression); **rigid mentality** gives rise to short-sightedness, impaired vision and hearing; **greed** makes us a slave to our bodily desires, etc. Do think it over!

3. What is the difference between soul pain and ego pain?

The needs of the ego are: attention, praise, admiration, recognition, acceptance, power and control over others. It is like a need to occupy the 'centre stage'.

The needs of our soul are: receptivity, keeping an open mind, perceiving a unity of purpose, honouring fellowship and going along with the needs of the larger system of which we are a part. These needs relate to the spiritual purpose of our life.

Ego pain is optional, you can let it go. *Soul pain* is NOT optional; either you correct it or you suffer.

4. How can we build our immunity to disease?

The two kinds of conflicts that are described above and the imbalance that results from them can be considered as the primary factors that generate our 'susceptibility' to illness. Hence, by logic, a person without these conflicts will have a natural immunity to illness.

The two basic errors can be termed as acts against our conscience, and acts against the principle of unity in society. And the remedial measures are to remove the thinking that generates these errors in our lifestyle and attitude. When we do that we have a 'talisman' against disease and also misfortune! In this way a 'diseased state' is preventable and curable.

5. How can we avoid the spread or increase of disease?

Orthodox medical science ignores the internal causes of disease. Instead, it tries to investigate the biological activity of all compounds that are discovered, both natural and synthetic, and it believes that someday it will find the remedies to eradicate disease from humanity! However, nature plays hide and seek with it. Nature generates newer and more resistant bacteria and newer diseases! This happens because the 'diseased state', which is a result of inner imbalance and conflict, is not overcome.

Thus, what the medicines can do indirectly for us we can do directly for ourselves! We can exercise our self-control and stop the thinking that extends the power of the diseased state in our nature. We can eliminate the specific defect or factor in our nature that creates our susceptibility to diseases and generate our immunity. And by acting in this way we can serve as an example for others. In this way we can spread the true message of health and healing.

Chapter-5:

Pranic Healing

Pranic Healing is an alternative to drug therapy that works on the holistic principle. It can be used to heal chronic ailments, internal organ troubles and psychosomatic disorders. It is most commonly used to treat exhaustion, congestions, backaches, and stress related disorders. Besides this, if anyone takes Pranic Healing treatment, they will instinctively understand the nature of the vital force in the energy (pranic) body.

To use Pranic Healing, the healer does not need to know the nature of a disease in detail. The cause of the ailment may be due to improper lifestyle like bad dietary or eating habits; excessive physical or emotional stress; improper medical treatment; or even a childhood trauma. However, the healer doesn't have to deal with these causes. He only deals with the effect these causes have had on the pranic (energy) body. The Pranic Healer does two things: He feels the condition of pranic energy in the body organs and restores the circulation of prana in the organs. Once the flow of prana is restored, the natural intelligence of the body does the healing. In this section we discuss what pranic healing can do for you and how you can learn to do pranic healing.

What Pranic Healing can do for you

1. What is pranic healing?

Generally speaking, an ailment arises in the body when its cells or organs are functioning improperly. And the disturbance in functioning happens due to an insufficient supply of prana or due to a congestion of spoilt prana in some part of the body. Hence, the treatment is to simply restore the flow of fresh prana in the body part. The healer first *drains out* the spoilt prana from the ailing part. Next, he *injects* some fresh prana in it. And then he restores the *circulation* of prana in the pranic body. As a result there is an increase in the supply of pranic energy to the part and better circulation of prana in the body. The usual effect of this treatment is that the patient begins to feel good very quickly.

The healer uses his hands to feel the prana at different places in the body. He feels the sensation of a blockage or a pull in certain areas. Where there is a blockage, it indicates that there is a congestion of corrupted prana in that area. Then draining out this prana becomes the most important step. Where there is a pull, it indicates that there is a deficiency of prana in that area. Then energising the area or organ with fresh prana becomes the most important step. Finally, the healer glides his hand over the area to restore the circulation of prana in the pranic body. Once the circulation is established, fresh prana will begin to flow to the organ or area. Then the vital force of the body will take over and perform the healing.

2. The nature of pranic energy

In Chinese this energy is called 'chi' and in Japanese it is called 'ki'. You can think of it as a subtle life-energy fluid. When the patient is open and receptive to this kind of treatment, this energy flows readily from the healer to the patient. However, if there is some resistance in the patient (due to fear, disbelief or protest) the flow of energy is restrained.

You can source the pranic energy in three ways: You can use the pranic energy that is in your body; you can generate it fresh as a vibration by chanting a mantra; or you can draw it from the atmosphere (its universal source). Beginners usually use their personal energy to perform the healing. However, if they do not generate the prana or learn to draw it from the greater source, they easily get exhausted. They feel drained or become irritable. So it is important for a healer to learn how to draw this energy from its universal source.

To be able to draw the pranic energy from the universal source, you have to become humble and call for it. When you are connected with this energy, you can feel it. Then you can channel it through you. However, when your mind is disturbed by negative thoughts or emotions, you get disconnected.

Although Pranic Healing is normally done with the hands, advanced healers can also transfer the prana psychically, through the gaze.

3. How pranic energy functions in the body

In addition to the physical body we have a 'pranic double-body'. It is a subtle body that extends to about three inches beyond the physical body. This double-body can absorb prana from inside and outside the body. However, its main function is to distribute the prana throughout the whole body. The prana also flows along certain channels, which are called 'nadis'. Most (not all) of the pranic channels run parallel to the nerve channels.

In addition to the energy currents, there are also energy centres or nodes within the pranic body. They are called 'chakras'. These chakras distribute the pranic energy to the endocrine glands and to the more subtle astral bodies. Hence, any deficiency of prana or congestion of spoilt prana in these chakras causes great imbalance in the person.

4. What the healer does

First, the healer will scan the body to detect the disturbance in the flow of the pranic energy currents. Next, he will cleanse the prana from the area where it is congested. Then, he will revitalise the area by giving fresh prana to it. After doing that he will re-establish the flow of prana and then close the energy field of the pranic body. The last step is necessary to ensure that the pranic currents continue to flow smoothly without getting dissipated or returning to the earlier condition.

In this way the healer can relieve the patient of many common ailments like colds, coughs, fevers, flu, headaches, backaches, muscle aches, joint pains, sprains, burns, fungus infections, etc.

5. Treating psychosomatic illnesses with pranic healing

Anger, fear, frustration, sorrow and negative thinking generate emotional entities on the astral plane. When you harbour such entities for a long time, they settle as parasites in your atmosphere and give rise to 'energy locks' in the pranic body. And these energy locks in time give rise to ailments in the physical body.

You can consider the emotional entities as personal thoughts with motives locked in. Modern psychotherapy tries to work with these emotional energies indirectly, whereas the Pranic Healer can work on them directly! The healer can draw out these entities from the astral body to release the energy locks in the pranic body. However, the patient has to collaborate in the process by willingly releasing the emotions. They have to give them up *without* holding on to them in the form of grudges or sentiments. When the patient holds on to the grudges or tries to justify them, the emotional entities will return. However, when the energy locks are released, the patient will be relieved from the phobias or obsessions that had kept them captive for years! Further, if there is some left over physical ailment, it will respond to any treatment.

For GENERAL CLEANING of the astral body: The treatment can be given in the standing, or sitting (on a stool), or a lying down position. First, the healer activates the energy in his hands to vibrate at the astral level. Next, he visualises large brushes of about two to three inches long coming out of his palms. Then he starts brushing the astral body in the downward direction, from head to the trunk. He brushes it both from the front and back and keeps on releasing the negative energy from his hands by flicking it out.

While doing this work he would normally ask the patient to *collaborate* with the healing process. The patient has to join in by visualising the negative energy being pulled out and thrown out. When the patient collaborates with the treatment, the healing becomes a surer process. The end result is that the patient feels lighter and released from emotional pressure after this treatment.

For treating deep emotional wounds like those that arise from abuse, personal loss, unresolved trauma or long-standing psychological troubles like fluctuating moods, the patient should seek the assistance of an advanced healer who has the power to treat the energy in the chakras.

6. The Chakras in Pranic Healing

The chakras are energy centres in the pranic double-body. They are somewhat aligned with the spine. When there is a disturbance in the energy field of a chakra, it disturbs the functioning of certain endocrine glands and gives rise to certain attitudes and psychological disturbances. Pranic healing can be used to clean the energy of a chakra and also enlarge and activate it. Many deep psychological conditions can be corrected in this way. In most patients the chakras will be small and so it may take some time in locating a chakra. Here we describe the chakras and the disturbances that can be corrected by treating them.

Here is an outline of some disorders that can be effectively treated by pranic healers:

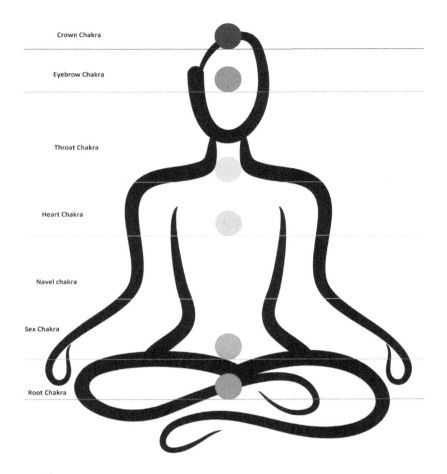

Crown Chakra

Eyebrow Chakra

Throat Chakra

Heart Chakra

Navel chakra

Sex Chakra

Root Chakra

a. The ROOT CHAKRA

When there is congestion of spoilt prana in the root chakra the person's basic support system is disturbed. There are survival or self-esteem issues, and the person may be considering the suicide option. Such effects can be relieved by treating this chakra. When it is properly done, it will totally change the disposition of the person. The treatment has to be followed up with some corrections in thinking and self-talk.

b. The SEX CHAKRA

When there is a congestion of spoilt prana in the sex chakra there is an imbalance in sensual desires. Some people develop gluttonous eating habits; some people experience uncontrollable sexual desire; and some others develop a strong desire to be appreciated. Lack of prana here would indicate that the person has lost his or her charm and perhaps also has some sexually related trouble. There may be a weakness in the ovaries, testicles, rectum, bladder or the small intestines. Excess energy in this chakra makes a person charming, but if this energy is not diverted to the higher chakras there is a tendency to drift towards perversion. Hence, this chakra has to be treated carefully to balance the energy here. There should be no deficiency or excess.

c. The NAVEL CHAKRA

When there is a lack of energy in this chakra, the person will lack self-confidence. He or she may have difficulty in asserting oneself. Such a person can easily get frustrated or recoil into a 'protest mode'. Deficiency of prana in this chakra is often associated with weakness in digestion. On the other hand, when there is excess prana here the person can easily become aggressive, manipulative or greedy. However, when the prana in this chakra is balanced, the person acts with confidence. There will be no tendency to bully or get bullied.

d. The HEART CHAKRA

This chakra is very sensitive to feelings. When a person is carrying an emotional hurt, the energy in this chakra will be less. A feeling of rejection, of being treated unjustly, or of being cheated drains away the energy of this chakra. The person feels not cared for, not valued or not loved and can become insensitive towards others. Excess energy in this chakra makes a person very demonstrative in their feelings. Sometimes they show a very vital behaviour. Whenever this chakra is properly energised, the person becomes peaceful, gentle and caring. He or she does not feel emotionally dependent on others.

e. The THROAT CHAKRA

This chakra governs our aesthetic sense and creative urges. When the energy of this chakra is balanced, the person has good expression, communication and creativity; and he or she is able to do meticulous work. When energy is lacking in this chakra, the person usually experiences frustration on some of these matters. A congestion of spoilt prana here can make a person talkative, worried or over-meticulous. It can also give rise to frequent ailments in the mouth, ears, nose, throat or neck.

f. The EYEBROW CHAKRA

This chakra governs the ability to do abstract and conceptual thinking and to exercise the will power. When this chakra is well developed, the person has psychic power (the sixth sense) – the power to command things, to heal, and to visualize and act on mental images. When there is a lack of energy in this chakra, the person has attention deficiency, is unable to conceptualise, and is unable to command things. In addition there can be weakness in the eyes, the pituitary gland and the lower brain. Many of these troubles can be relieved by activating this chakra through practices like tratak (steady gazing). Pranic healing can be used to give 'finishing effects'.

g. The CROWN CHAKRA

This chakra has a bearing on our connection with the over-soul or the universal consciousness. A well developed crown chakra makes a person naturally intuitive and dharmic. When there is a lack of energy in this chakra the person is disconnected from the higher consciousness. Such a person can easily develop atheistic tendencies, feel purposeless, or lack the dharma sense. He or she will keep on looking for solutions in the wrong places! Such disturbances cannot be healed through persuasion, but they can be corrected by energising this chakra.

7. The treatment

The healer usually dips his hand into the energy field of the chakra and begins to *weed out* the negative energy from it. He draws it out and flicks it away. After cleaning the energy field, he *injects* some fresh prana into the chakra. He may do it by chanting a mantra and waving his hand over the area of the chakra. He may also try to enlarge the chakra by spreading its energy over a slightly wider the area.

If the healer needs to have an *intense effect* on a chakra, he will keep his right hand at the back of the chakra (spine) and the left hand on the front side. Then he will push the energy from the right hand through the chakra into the left hand.

After treating one or more chakras, the healer will *balance* the flow of energy inside the spinal cord that connects the chakras. He will push the energy up and down to clear the blockages in the flow of energy. This is done to ensure that the chakra remains replenished. In addition, if there is a congestion of excess prana in the lower chakras, the energy will be profitably diverted to energise some of the higher chakras. In this connection it is interesting to note some of the connections of the lower chakras with the higher chakras. In particular, the second chakra is connected with the fifth chakra. So, the sexual force can be diverted to enhance the aesthetic side of the person. In the same way, the third chakra is connected with the sixth chakra. Hence, energy from desires and ambition can be diverted to strengthen the central will-force. In the same way, the fourth and seventh chakras are connected. Hence, devotional practices can develop the truth sense and soul power.

Clearing the blockages in flow of inter-chakra energy also has great value for persons who are doing spiritual practice. It can show them what parts of them are progressing too fast and what parts are lagging behind. If the imbalance is allowed to continue, they become prone to illness.

After cleaning, charging, and balancing the chakras, the healer will *close* the energy field. It ensures that the effect of the healing continues for some time.

This work on a chakra is usually done in small portions at a time. It gives the patient the time they need to make the adjustments in their attitude and lifestyle to be able to sustain the new energy field.

8. Self-Healing using prana

Sit in a chair with eyes closed and visualise the pranic energy as a glow of white light over the crown of your head. If you cannot visualise it properly, just think that it is there.

Next, begin to draw the light down into your body. Do it as follows: First let it enter the brain, then the face, and then gradually let it come down into the chest and the belly. Ultimately let it flow into the feet. As the light comes down, try to feel that it is spreading into the cells of the organs and pushing out the corrupted prana. Do the exercise slowly. If your attention lapses during the exercise, start again from where you slipped off.

In the end visualise (see with eyes closed) that your whole body is filled with a soft-white pranic light. Try to feel the calm and peace. Persist with this exercise for a few months and it will not only refresh you, but it will also relieve many of your physical and emotional ailments.

Learning to do pranic healing

1. Sensitizing the hands

Although anyone can receive prana, if you want to become a healer you have to first sensitise your hands. The process of developing healing hands is more of an art than a science. It takes more time for some people and less time for others. The ability to heal also varies greatly from person to person.

Normally you begin the process by sensitizing the *finger tips*. At least the first three fingers of each hand should be sensitised. The method is simple. Put some mustard seeds in the palm of one hand and try to sense them with a finger of the other hand. Do this practice daily until you can count the number of seeds accurately.

Next, place a hair or wire between two sheets of paper and try to sense it by slowly gliding your fingers over the paper. Then learn to recognise some small objects by feeling them without looking at them. Continue such practices for a few weeks and you will have developed the necessary sensitivity in your fingers.

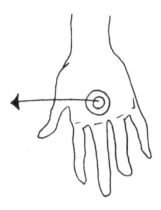

Then you can go further and activate the chakra in the *palm* of your hands. Place the index finger of the right hand on the left palm and move it in the clockwise direction. Then pass energy from the finger into the palm and try to feel the energy passing through. Then place the index finger of the left hand on the right palm and move it in the anticlockwise direction. Then pass energy from the finger and try to sense the energy current. After you can do this, repeat these exercises by keeping the finger at a distance of one inch from the palm.

Next, try to feel the energy *between the palms* of your two hands from a distance of 1 inch to 1 foot. Keep the hands at a distance of 1 inch and bring energy into them. Then feel the energy as you separate them slowly up to one foot. Now keep the hands one foot away and feel the energy between the hands. Then move them close together and feel the energy being compressed. During these exercises, try to feel the warmth, the tingling, the magnetism, the pull and the compression.

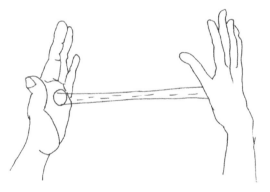

After you have done this preparation for a few months, sit opposite a person who has healing hands and pass the energy from your right hand into his left hand and from his right hand into your left hand. It will open up the hand chakras sufficiently and give you the power to do pranic healing. This ability will develop further as you use it.

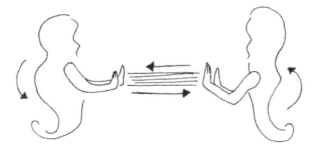

Many people regard pranic healing as a subject for research. They make claims to have found something new and try to develop their 'personal brand' around it. However, the truth is that pranic healing is as old as humanity; and it needs no development! It is for individuals to develop their personal ability so that they can use it effectively. The ability to heal does not depend so much on learning the technique, but it depends more on the spiritual power of the healer.

2. Sensing the patient's energy field

First have the patient remove silk, rubber, leather, and metal items from their body. Then ask them to lie down on a cot. Now hold your left hand steady at a distance of about two to five inches above the person's head (body) and gently glide the right hand down. Feel the pranic currents in the patient's body as the hand goes down. Here is a brief description of what you may sense:

- Sensation of heat in an area may indicate a congestion of emotions like anger
- Sensation of cold may indicate emotions like fear
- A pull of the energy from your hand indicates a deficiency of prana in the area
- A magnetic block (resistance) indicates an accumulation of spoilt prana
- Sensation of dullness or roughness indicates an accumulation of negative energy.

3. Giving the treatment

First, make some slow passes over the (pranic) body. Keep your left hand over the patient's head and slowly glide your right hand over the affected areas in the patient's body. Focus your attention on draining out the negative energy from the sensitive areas as completely as possible. The spoilt prana can be pulled out with the right hand. The stroking should be done in the downward (from head down) or outward (from the trunk out) direction. The corrupted prana that you draw out has to be thrown out. You can do it by shaking or flicking your hand.

Both the healer and the patient should be able to feel the negative energy that is being drawn out. In case of minor injuries, it may only take a few seconds to draw out the energy. In major illnesses or chronic troubles it can take more time, and you can only draw out a little at a time. Hence, the treatment has to be given over a few sessions.

After you have drawn out the negative energy, you can tell the patient that you are going to put in positive energy. Then point the right hand over the sensitive area and pump in the energy by willing it. Gently pass it on by waving your hand over it. You can ask the patient to feel the energy that is flowing in. After sufficient energy has been put in, smooth out the energy by spreading it over a slightly wider area.

Then you have to close the energy field. You do it by simply willing the prana to stay as you make a pass over the patient's body with your right hand. When this is properly done, the healing will continue for hours and sometimes for days after the treatment. You can follow this procedure for treating most acute and chronic troubles.

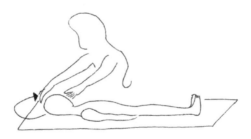

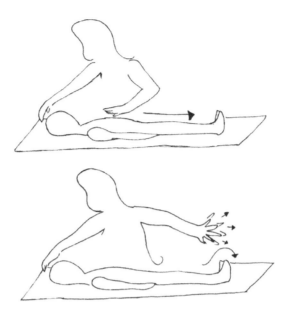

4. What to expect after the treatment

Your treatment will bring about a shift in the energy level in the patient. When the blockages in the flow of pranic energy have been removed and fresh prana has been injected into the system the patient will feel energised. You should allow the person to remain lying down for a few minutes to let the energy settle in. The person will leave the session feeling good.

Once the body is energised, you can expect the healing to continue for some time – sometimes for a few days. Often the healing can be completed only to an extent in one session. Then you have to call the patient for another session to complete the healing. Long standing troubles can require treatment over many sessions spread over a few weeks.

5. How to end the healing session

You should end a session smoothly and not abruptly. Think that you are nurturing the patient and not abandoning him. So, at the end of a session, tell the patient: *"Your body is healing. We have initiated the process and the body knows what to do. Your body will continue to heal for some time".* This suggestion will help the patient so that the healing can continue for a longer time after the session

Immediately after giving the healing treatment allow the patient to rest for some time. They should not straight away get up and walk out. In this way they give the body some time to adjust to the change in the energy field.

You can ask the patient to increase the water intake for a few days after taking the treatment. It will assist the natural cleansing of the body. Also ask the patient not to wash the treated parts with water for the next 12 hours. The washing can drain away some of the immediate effect of the treatment.

Sometimes there may be a short 'healing crisis' after the treatment. The patient feels better, but some symptoms get aggravated. Some discharges or the body temperature may increase. The patient should consider such symptoms as a part of the natural cleansing process and not suppress these symptoms (discharges or fever) with drugs or medicated ointments.

6. Care in discharging the negative prana

As a healer you can often pick up negative prana from the patients you treat. Hence, you should take care to release this energy quickly and completely. You can do it by washing your hands with water and by imagining the negative energy as being washed away. The people who do regular pranic healing usually dip their hands into salt water and then rinse them with fresh water to clear all the negative energy clinging to their fingers.

If water is not available, you can discharge the negative energy by gently rubbing the hands on the floor (earth) or by vigorously flicking the energy out of the fingers while directing them to the earth.

What happens if you don't clear the negative energy after the session? It can leave you feeling sluggish or drained out. In psychological disorders the negative energy can disturb you emotionally.

If you are practising pranic healing regularly, you should also clear the negative energy from your working area. You can do it by chanting a mantra and directing the vibrating energy through your hand into the environment.

7. Distance healing

Distance healing is giving treatment from a long distance. Here the prana is sent as a *'mental vibration'*, like a mantra, to the patient. You direct it to the patient through a 'mental image'.

First, you make a mental image of the patient. Next, you visualise it sufficiently to establish a connection between the image and the energy body of the patient. Then, you clear the energy channels mentally; transmit the prana directly into the sensitive area in the organ; and then close the energy field to allow the healing to continue. You do all this with your gaze. The patient will feel a warm sensation while receiving the prana.

There are advantages and disadvantages to this method. In present healing the patient feels your presence and can collaborate in the healing process. It gives him the faith that it will work out; and you get the feedback and feel enthusiastic. In distance healing the patient does not feel your presence and you don't get the necessary feedback. Further, in distant healing it is easy to put in the prana, but it is not so easy to draw out the spoilt prana. The main advantage of distance healing is convenience to the patient. The healer also has the advantage of not being distracted by the presence of other people that may be around.

Generally speaking, when you undertake to heal, it is requested by the patient. Then there is openness and trust. In distance healing, however, the request is usually made indirectly by a family member or a friend. The patient may be in a 'denial mode', wherein he or she is unwilling to acknowledge the cause or is psychologically not receptive to this kind of healing. Then if you push the prana into the person, the resistance can spoil the quality of the prana and cause disturbance in both the patient and the healer. Hence, my suggestion is that indirect requests for healing should not be accepted. Further, you should limit the use of the distant healing only to follow up on your 'present healing' cases.

Appendix

About the Author

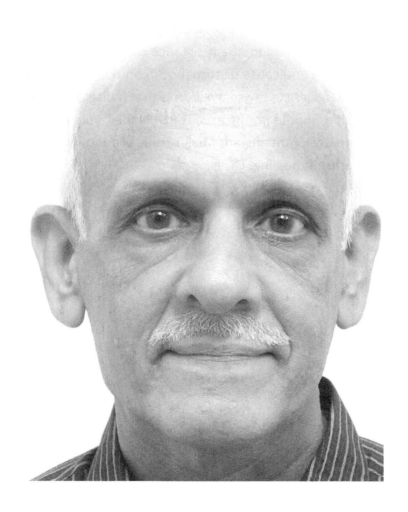

Prashant S. Shah was educated in Chemistry from Massachusetts Institute of Technology (BS, MIT, USA) and

University of California at Santa Cruz (MS, PhC, UCSC, USA). He learnt Mysticism from Shri Nyaya Sharma, a Master of Shiva Tantra Yoga and Homoeopathy from Post Graduate Homoeopathic Association, Bombay. He has healing hands and uses Pranic Healing. This book is an outcome of his personal experience of over 40 years.

He has worked as a scientist, a businessman, a management consultant, a counsellor, and a spiritual guide. He conducts correspondence courses for implementing spiritual practice through Darshana Centre, a school of mysticism at Baroda. He is the Author of many books and a Speaker at many spiritual awareness programs. He speaks clearly, in simple language, and from personal experience. Other books written and published by the author are:

- *How to Restore your Health Naturally (2017)*
- *The Biochemic Prescriber (2016)*
- *Solving the Problems of Life (2015)*
- *The Art of Awakening the Soul (2011)*
- *The Practice of Mysticism (2009)*
- *Essence of Hindu Astrology (1987)*
- *Crisis of Modern Humanity (1976)*

For more information on the books, articles and workshops by the author visit the site on Internet at http://spiritual-living.in

Other books by the Author

1. The Biochemic Prescriber

A guide for prescribing Dr. Schuessler's biochemic tissue salts to family and friends

92 pages. ISBN-13: 978-1533128065; ISBN-10: 1533128065
ASIN: B01FA6X4FG

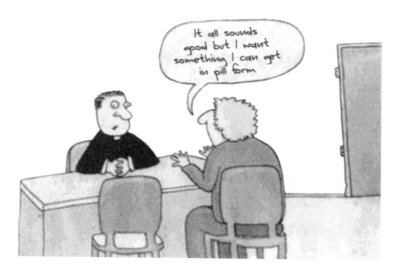

We have often been confronted with questions like these. The patient just wants relief from a particular ailment. Sometimes it is only a temporary functional disorder. And for all such troubles we have a very good solution:

It avoids the drug therapy, but uses vibrated sugar pills instead. Hence, there are no side-effects or after-effects. It is easy to diagnose your ailment by noting the 'guiding symptoms'. With a little familiarity it is easy to use or prescribe. And the remedies, the vibrated sugar pills are readily available from the market! To know more, read our little book on the Biochemic System.

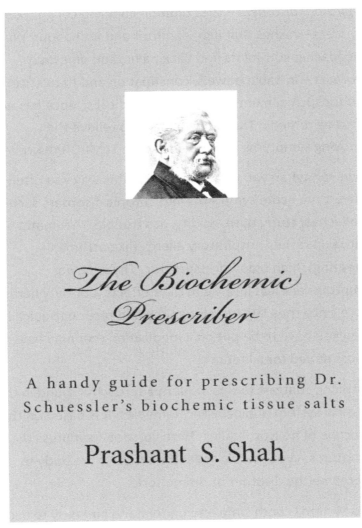

The Biochemic Prescriber

A handy guide for prescribing Dr. Schuessler's biochemic tissue salts

Prashant S. Shah

Allopathic medicine is the mainstream system. It is a leader for treatment in emergencies, in infectious diseases, and for ailments that require surgical intervention. However, most of the common troubles that we face are only FUNCTIONAL DISORDERS, such as: *respiratory disorders* – the common cold and cough; *skin disorders* – rashes that itch, dandruff and foul odour; *pains* – headache, stiff-joints and back pains; and *digestive disorders* – irritable bowels, constipation and flatulence. And for such ailments the modern medical science has no effective remedy. They only manage to relieve the annoying symptoms and provide some TEMPORARY relief.

However, when you treat the body in this way you often convert the acute symptoms into chronic disorders such as headaches, stuffy nose, acidity, gas trouble, rheumatic pain, skin rashes, respiratory allergy (like asthma, wheezing), high blood pressure, etc. These newer symptoms are less intense in their effects, but they harass more since they last for a long time and recur periodically. Then you have to be put on a medication that may have to be continued for a lifetime!

A striking contrast to this modern approach is found in the classical system of Biochemic Remedies. It is based on the principle of holistic healing. Here you don't suppress the symptoms – you merely assist the effort of the body to overcome the disorder or discomfort.

This system is both simple to understand and easy to use. And it comes without the 'side-effects' that usually arise from using the drug therapy. The most interesting thing about this approach to healing is that you don't need to know in detail the functions of the body organs, the classification of disease, or have to rely on laboratory tests to be able to prescribe. My mother used to treat us (family) with these biochemic remedies when we were kids. And she did a pretty good job with it even though she had no training in healthcare!

To treat the patient effectively, you have to only study the 'guiding symptoms' indicated for each of the 12 biochemic remedies. I have personally used these biochemic remedies and over the years I have found the results to be consistent and very satisfactory.

This book is written from experience. Great care is taken to characterise the signature of each of the tissue-salts. You can use this short description to identify the remedy. It will save you a lot of time and effort. You have to take care to prescribe on the basis of the specific indications for these biochemic remedies and not on the basis of classified diseases.

With a little practice you can *become a domestic physician* (not a licensed physician). Then you can safely help yourself, your family and your friends in health matters. It will overcome your helplessness and reduce your dependence on the medical profession.

The book is available from **Amazon** and **Kindle online bookstores**. Use this handy prescriber to heal yourself, your family and friends. The treatment is simple to understand and easy to use; and the results are very consistent and satisfying.

Kindle online store: https://www.amazon.com/Biochemic-Prescriber-prescribing-Schusslers-biochemic-ebook/dp/B01FA6X4FG/
Amazon online store:
http://www.amazon.com/Biochemic-Prescriber-prescribing-Schussler-biochemic/dp/1533128065

2. The Art of Awakening the Soul

Yoga Mysticism

143 pages, ISBN-13: 978-1460906033, ISBN-10: 1460906039, ASIN: BOOAX19BRW; URL is http://www.amazon.com/dp/B00AXI9BRW/

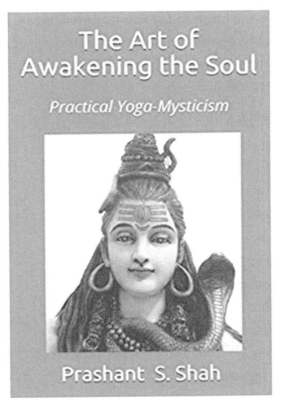

In this book you learn the practical art of attuning your mind with a higher consciousness. Then instead of being guided by the tendencies in your mind, you will be guided by a higher consciousness

This practice will gradually bring the soul forward in your life. The soul is your inner companion and it will give you the experience of deep love that cannot be got through the people and things of the outer world.

When the soul is sufficiently awake in your life, it will guide you, inform you, and make you intuitive. Then everything in your life will begin to fall into its proper place: You will know what to do with your life and your time; you will get the opportunities you really need; and the rest will not matter very much.

The Contents:

1. Foreword by the Author
2. What is Mysticism?
3. The Practice
4. The Basic Task
5. The Inner Work
6. The Practical Side of Purification
7. The Transformation
8. The Message
9. Aphorisms for Awakening
10. A Prayer
11. A Conversation
12. Articles:
13. Moments of Overflowing
14. A Journey into the Higher Worlds
15. Spiritual Alchemy
16. The Coming of the New Era

3. Solving the Problems of Life

For Spiritual Seekers

132 pages; ISBN-13: 9781518786655; ISBN-10: 1518786650; ASIN: B0176HQSOG. The URL is http://www.amazon.com/dp/B0176HQSOG

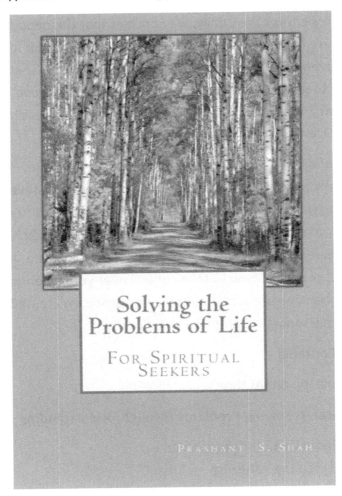

It is said that ships are safe in the harbour. But that is not what ships are made for. They are there so that we can sail through the rough seas and visit distant lands. In the same way we can suffer our problems and seek to avoid them; or we can treat them as opportunities to grow and enjoy the problem-solving process. *What will it be?*

When we think spiritually, we consider that the people who are involved with us and the happenings of our life are given to us. They provide us the opportunities that we need to grow. Just as a car needs the ground to move forward, a bird needs the air to fly, we need the resistance from life (the problems) to grow and mature.

This book will take you on a problem-solving journey. The journey passes through three chapters. First, you develop the right attitude towards your problems and life situation. Next, you go further and learn what you can do right now to experience freedom and contentment in your life. And lastly, you learn how to take control over your attention, and then you use it to overcome the problems created by your personal thoughts and emotions.

The Contents

Preface, by the Author

Chapter-1: Solving Problems through Understanding

1. Understand the trials of life
2. Lessen the suffering
3. Find guidance

4. Use understanding
5. Consider yourself as something special
6. Be optimistic
7. Be wise
8. Do not create problems for yourself
9. Overcome your inner enemies
10. Seek counsel
11. Don't ask for blessings, count your blessings
12. The school of life

Chapter-2: The Key to Freedom & Contentment

1. Accept what you cannot change
2. Freedom and how to achieve it
3. Approach life as a banquet
4. Act well the part that is given to you
5. All advantages have their price
6. Our duties are revealed by our relationships
7. Control your interpretations
8. Serve the greater purpose

Chapter-3: The Marvel of Mantra Yoga

a) Spiritual Yoga

1. Introduction
2. How do you begin?
3. Observing the mind — an illustration
4. Overcoming the drifting tendency
5. What exactly is concentration?
6. The practice

7. On Mantra Yoga
8. The key idea of Yoga
9. Is Spiritual Yoga theistic or atheistic?

b) Using Mantra Yoga

1. My introduction to mantra
2. My first benefits
3. The mantra tradition
4. The practice
5. Our personal or seminal sound
6. How chanting alters our personal vibration
7. Should you begin the practice with chanting or meditation?
8. Is the practice of meditation in mantra yoga theistic or atheistic?

c) On controlling Thoughts and Emotions

1. Dealing with intruding thoughts?
2. Dealing with troublesome thoughts
3. How do emotions arise?
4. Dealing with negative emotions
5. Clearing negative emotions

4. How to Restore your Health Naturally

A time-tested way to heal yourself by simply changing your lifestyle and eating habits

ISBN-13: 978-1977555472; ISBN-10: 1977555470; ASIN: B075V5R1FJ

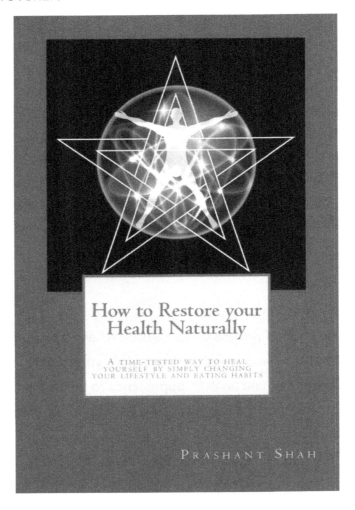

How to Restore your Health Naturally

A TIME-TESTED WAY TO HEAL YOURSELF BY SIMPLY CHANGING YOUR LIFESTYLE AND EATING HABITS

PRASHANT SHAH

Today we are ingrained to believe that our health depends on doctors, medicines, and the health care industry; whereas the truth is that our health really depends on our lifestyle, diet and emotions. When we understand this simple truth, we can learn to restore and maintain our health by our own efforts and, except in extreme cases, we will not need to consult doctors.

The method of natural healing that we show is holistic and totally different from the specialised advice that you normally receive through the medical profession. It is simple, and to use it you do not need to know anatomy, physiology, pathology, toxicology or pharmacology. Further, the results of this treatment are self-evident, and so you do not have to depend on empirical proofs. You simply strengthen the vital force in the body and help it in its effort to restore your health and keep you healthy.

Contents:

1. Foreword
2. Introduction
3. The medical profession focuses on relieving symptoms
4. What is so wrong with just relieving symptoms?
5. The holistic and analytic approaches to healing
6. Understanding disease in terms of toxaemia and the vital force
7. Aren't germs and bacteria the causes of disease?
8. How to detoxify the body
9. Reduce the existing toxaemia

© 2014-18, Prashant S. Shah

10. Avoid generating toxins
11. Correct your eating habits
12. On emotional causes
13. What causes the vital force to become weak?
14. The elimination crisis
15. If natural healing is so simple, why isn't everyone doing it?
16. Our message

Made in the USA
Middletown, DE
02 January 2024

47036637R00099